Population Health Science

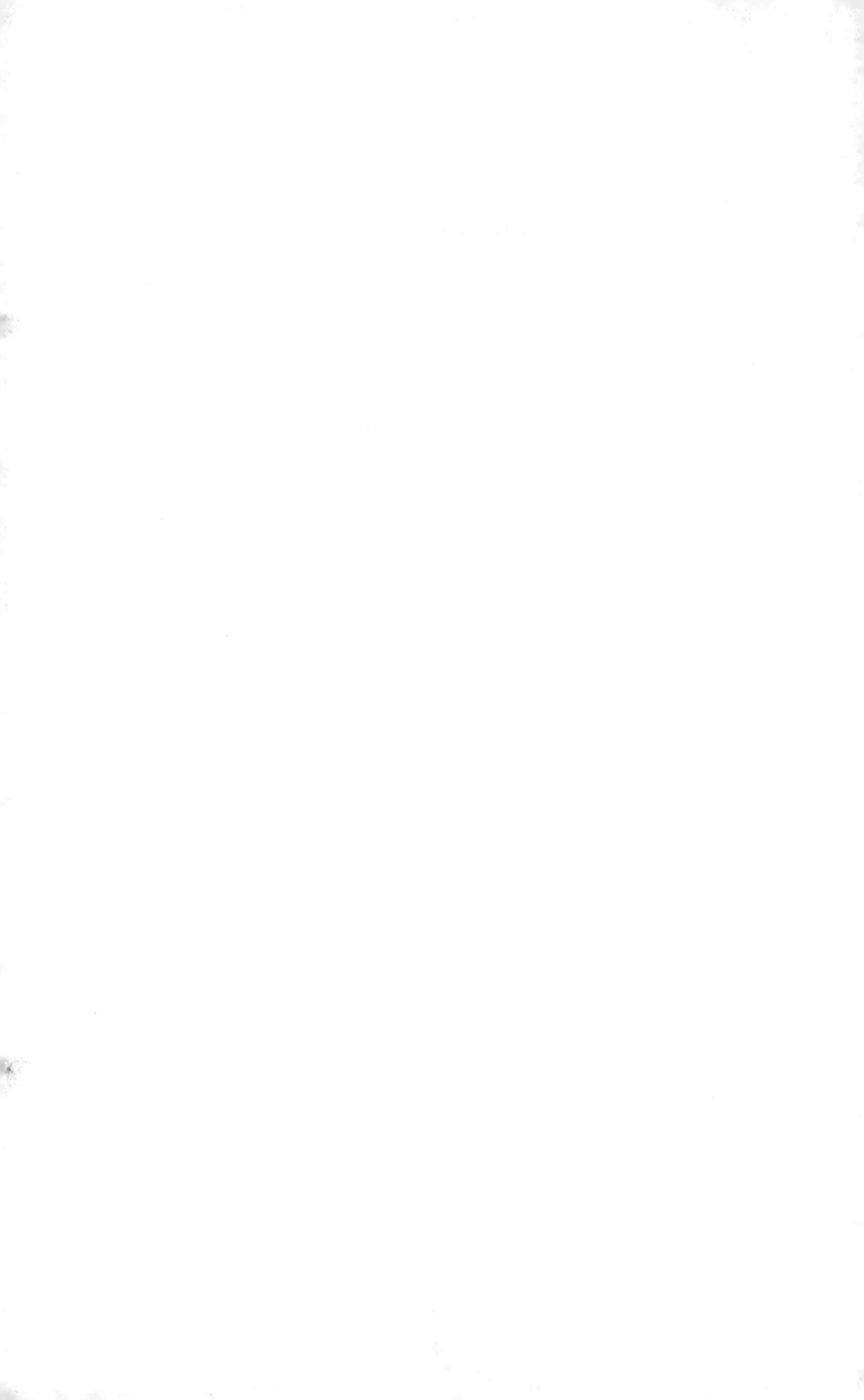

POPULATION HEALTH SCIENCE

KATHERINE M. KEYES

SANDRO GALEA

OXFORD
UNIVERSITY PRESS

OXFORD
UNIVERSITY PRESS

Oxford University Press is a department of the University of Oxford. It furthers the University's objective of excellence in research, scholarship, and education by publishing worldwide. Oxford is a registered trade mark of Oxford University Press in the UK and certain other countries.

Published in the United States of America by Oxford University Press
198 Madison Avenue, New York, NY 10016, United States of America.

© Oxford University Press 2016

All rights reserved. No part of this publication may be reproduced, stored in a retrieval system, or transmitted, in any form or by any means, without the prior permission in writing of Oxford University Press, or as expressly permitted by law, by license, or under terms agreed with the appropriate reproduction rights organization. Inquiries concerning reproduction outside the scope of the above should be sent to the Rights Department, Oxford University Press, at the address above.

You must not circulate this work in any other form
and you must impose this same condition on any acquirer.

Library of Congress Cataloging-in-Publication Data
Names: Keyes, Katherine M., author. | Galea, Sandro, author.
Title: Population health science / Katherine M. Keyes, Sandro Galea.
Description: Oxford ; New York : Oxford University Press, [2016]
Identifiers: LCCN 2016002636 (print) | LCCN 2016003088 (ebook) |
ISBN 9780190459376 (pbk. : alk. paper) | ISBN 9780190459383 (ebook) |
ISBN 9780190459390 (ebook)
Subjects: | MESH: Social Medicine—methods | Health Status | Health Status Indicators | Epidemiologic Methods
Classification: LCC RA407 (print) | LCC RA407 (ebook) | NLM WA 31 |
DDC 614.4/2—dc23
LC record available at http://lccn.loc.gov/2016002636

We dedicate this book to the memory and legacy of Geoffrey Rose, whose insights laid the foundation for population health science.

Contents

Acknowledgments ix
About the Authors xi
Foundational Principles of Population Health Science xiii

1. An Introduction to Population Health Science   1
2. Conceptualizing and Evaluating Causes for Population Health Science   13
3. The Causes of Cases Versus Causes of Incidence   25
4. Population Health Across Levels, Systems, and the Life Course   45
5. Ubiquity and the Macrosocial Determinants of Population Health   67
6. Causal Architecture to Understand What Matters Most: Theory   85
7. Causal Architecture and What Matters Most: Quantitative Examples   99
8. Valuing Population Health Interventions: Measuring Return on Investment   111
9. Equity and Efficiency in Population Health Science   129
10. Prediction in Population Health Science   141

11. Case Study: Can We Reduce Obesity by Encouraging People to Eat Healthy Food?   157

12. Case Study: Simulating the Impact of High-Risk and Population Intervention Strategies for the Prevention of Disease   171

13. Tensions in Population Health Science   191

Index   203

Acknowledgments

WRITING THIS BOOK could not have been done without the support and assistance of an excellent team. We are indebted to the editorial assistance of Angelina Casazza, who provided review and synthesis of literature, critical edits, and superb translation of often poorly drawn, hand-written graphs. Ava Hamilton also assisted with graphs and figures. Caroline Rutherford provided assistance with our numerical examples, catching many of our errors along the way. All remaining errors are ours alone.

Jonathan Platt, doctoral student in epidemiology at Columbia University, collaborated with us on two chapters in this volume, working tirelessly through many iterations. His keen insights on population health science and simulation were immensely helpful. Gregory Cohen, also a doctoral student in epidemiology at Columbia University, generously contributed to our example of multilevel causes of cardiovascular disease.

We gained valuable clarification from a meeting held at Boston University on the topic of population health science attended by Jennifer Ahern, Jacob Bor, Greg Cohen, Catherine Ettman, Atheendar Venkataramani, Laura Sampson, Daniel Westreich, and Joana Lima.

Chad Zimmerman has been an excellent editor, providing support and encouragement, humor, and a keen eye all along the way.

Finally, we thank our families and loved ones for allowing us the time to write this volume, including evenings, weekends, and even vacations. This book would not be possible without their unwavering support.

About the Authors

Katherine M. Keyes, PhD, is Assistant Professor of Epidemiology at the Columbia University Mailman School of Public Health, New York City.

Sandro Galea, MD, DrPH, is Dean and Robert A. Knox Professor at the Boston University School of Public Health, Boston.

Foundational Principles of Population Health Science

1. Population health manifests as a continuum.
2. The causes of differences in health across populations are not necessarily an aggregate of the causes of differences in health within populations.
3. Large benefits to population health may not improve the lives of all individuals.
4. The causes of population health are multilevel, accumulate throughout the life course, and are embedded in dynamic interpersonal relationships.
5. Small changes in ubiquitous causes may result in more substantial change in the health of populations than larger changes in rarer causes.
6. The magnitude of an effect of exposure on disease is dependent on the prevalence of the factors that interact with that exposure.
7. Prevention of disease often yields a greater return on investment than curing disease after it has started.
8. Efforts to improve overall population health may be a disadvantage to some groups; whether equity or efficiency is preferable is a matter of values.
9. We can predict health in populations with much more certainty than we can predict health in individuals.

1

An Introduction to Population Health Science

POPULATION HEALTH SCIENCE is the study of the conditions that shape distributions of health within and across populations, and of the mechanisms through which these conditions manifest in the health of individuals. Population health science is hitting its stride; several leading schools of public health are launching doctoral programs in population health science, and trainees in these schools are increasingly considering themselves population health scientists. But what is *population health science*? Is it simply public health in a new cloak? To us, population health science is, simply, the science of the health of populations. As a science, it generates, tests, and confirms or rejects hypotheses about the causes of health states in populations. As a pragmatic science, it aims to do so in a way that we may marshal evidence as a means to inform policies, programs, and interventions that improve the health of populations. In this book, we present foundations of population health science to provide readers and the field with formative core principles around which we can organize our thinking and scholarship. In this first chapter we outline the motivation for this text; provide our definitions and assumptions about populations, health, and science; and articulate the first foundational principle of a science of population health.

1.0 The Motivation and Foundation for This Text

We are at a particularly important juncture in the field of population health. After a century with critical wins for public health (Centers for Disease Control and Prevention 2013)—including the development of sanitation and clean-water efforts, critical vaccines for the reduction of childhood morbidity and mortality, widespread work promoting smoking cessation, reductions in traffic fatality through consumer safety efforts, and massive undertakings to reduce mother-to-child and other human immunodeficiency virus (HIV) transmission worldwide—we are faced increasingly with challenging chronic and acute diseases for which no clear answers are apparent. Academic research on how to solve these problems—focused now, more than ever, on the methods we use— often hits a wall, yielding few answers that have the potential to move the needle on population health. On the positive side, creative strategies from across disciplines are being applied to pressing public health problems. For example, we have recently seen approaches from behavioral economics and computer science introduced to population health, with promising early results (Rice 2013; Zinszer et al. 2015).

This, then, is a propitious time. As the diseases that yielded public health victories during the 20th century fade away, we are faced with complex diseases, some emergent and some that have always placed a burden on population health, which shall require our ingenuity and versatility. They shall also require clarity about what we do, about what we aspire to achieve in population health science, and how we may get there. This book aims to be a marker along the road to get there. We charge readers with first considering the principles of what a science of population health should be, and how we go about asking questions about population health—framing research that matters and is consequential—and understanding the foundational principles of population health science.

The time is right for such articulation. Despite decades of solid empirical work in the domain of population health science and across disciplinary boundaries from demography, sociology, anthropology, psychology, epidemiology, economics, and other fields, there remains little consensus on the goals and foundational principles that govern the conduct of population health science. Perhaps the closest we have come to such an articulation is in Geoffrey Rose's volume *The Strategy of Preventive Medicine*, published more than two decades ago (Rose 1992). Our field has progressed rapidly since that time, however, with emerging epidemics of both infectious and chronic disease challenging us to create new paradigms of scientific inquiry and to develop technologies in data collection, storage, and use, allowing us unparalleled ability to test hypotheses that had not even been considered in previous decades.

This volume owes a large debt to Geoffrey Rose who, in our assessment, did seminal work in articulating the early foundational principles of population health science. Here, with due humility, we aim to extend his work, incorporating new insights that have emerged during the past two decades, and to demarcate the boundaries of a new population health science for a new generation of scholars. Although we discuss methods that are appropriate for analyzing research questions of interest to population health, this is not a methodological text. Our central purpose is to articulate and expand on principles that allow readers to engage in population health thinking, and to have a platform and reservoir of theory from which to draw when formulating questions of relevance to population health.

We note that although our work is informed explicitly by *A Strategy for Preventive Medicine* (Rose 1992), we adopt a broader lens. We do so not to negate the role of prevention or prevention science, but rather because we have come to see prevention as part of a broader armamentarium of efforts to improve the health of populations, some that are preventive and some that aim to improve population disease profiles. We suggest the principles we articulate here are equally applicable to a prevention science agenda, but are broader than that. These principles are grounded in an understanding of populations and how we can improve health in populations both before and after disease occurs. We note in particular chapters of this book when the lessons we discuss have bearing on prevention; but, in many ways, all the areas we cover are informative for our understanding of prevention and the science thereof. We leave it to others to build off our work to improve on the strategy of preventive medicine proposed by Rose directly.

We believe population health science represents a way of thinking, rather than a particular set of questions or methods. As such, in this book we approach population health science theoretically; we walk readers through foundational principles of the field while broadly discussing different methodological approaches to addressing questions of population health relevance. We took this approach for two reasons. First, there has not been, to our knowledge, an articulation of the principles of population health science in the modern era. As our field has grown, diversified, and incorporated theory and methods from across different disciplines, the time is right for a consolidation of the principles that guide us as population health researchers. Second, a presentation of particular methods applicable to population health science would constitute many more than one volume of text. A thorough understanding of biostatistics and study design are necessary for any population health scientist, however these are necessary but insufficient foundations to engage in population health research. We opt, instead, to provide a platform for how to think in terms of populations and present suggested principles of population health science as an organizing framework for a quickly growing field.

2.0 What Is a Population?

To start thinking in terms of population health, we first must consider what we mean when we say *population*. Typically, we think of populations as collections of people or other organisms that share common characteristics, most often a specific location they inhabit. Thus, the population of a specific town, village, city, state, or country is all those who live within that geographically defined boundary. Populations can also be defined by other organizing characteristics, such as individuals who are eligible for enrollment in a specific kind of study, women who are pregnant in a given year in a specific geographic area, or individuals with a specific medical condition. Thus, the two conditions to be a population are (1) there is more than one individual and (2) these individuals share at least one common characteristic.

There are two aspects of populations that are important to consider as we progress toward conceptualizing population health science. First, populations are almost always dynamic. Individuals move in and out of geographic locations, grow older, die, move in and out of health states, and vary across time, in terms of exposure levels, to acute and chronic exposures. Thus, most populations are moving targets. At any moment in time, the composition of a population is changing.

Second, we define the population of interest based on a number of considerations that include those of scientific or public health interest. That is, we may be concerned with the health of the population of a specific city if we work for the health department of that city, or we may be concerned with the health of a certain country because it has a particularly high burden of disease. But, we define the boundaries of what a population of interest is to us based on characteristics such as place, time, and person, as well as eligibility criteria. Thus, there is nothing inherently sacrosanct and constant about populations; they are constantly shifting and moving in terms of composition, and are defined based on our interests as researchers or practitioners. This situation agitates for clarity about the populations with which we are concerned, and flexibility of perspective regarding how we may analyze these populations.

3.0 What Is Science and What Is Population Health Science?

Science is a process that involves establishing theory from observation; creating hypotheses from these theories; testing these hypotheses using data in ways that allow us to refute, refine, or specify a theory; and moving forward in the progression of creating an evidence base for action. In concept, population health science is no different than other sciences. We are concerned centrally with understanding how the health of populations is produced. We formulate hypotheses about causes and effects, and about the changes we might expect if we manipulate one particular input or another. We design our studies to test these hypotheses, proving or disproving them, with the aim of informing the practice of public health.

An understanding of the epistemology of science, however, is particularly relevant to population health science. The philosophy of science has built a wealth of theory that guides how we ask a research question, accumulate evidence, test hypotheses, and move our science forward (e.g., Popper 1959). This same body of scholarship teaches us, however, that "truth" in science is an abstract concept. Scholars such as Ludwik Fleck (1981) noted in the early 20th century that researchers and scientists form "thought collectives" that reinforce each other, such that any truth generated from science is not absolute, but rather relative, informed by the collective thinking through which the question itself emerges. This idea has been linked to scholarship further investigating how we approach our science, among authors such as Kuhn (1962) and, more broadly, Foucault (1982), who have argued that as scientists we form collective beliefs and assumptions about causal (and noncausal) relationships that form paradigms of thought and lines of inquiry. These paradigms shift periodically and cyclically as neglected lines of inquiry and forms of thought become rediscovered. Thus, the progression of science is nonlinear; our research questions are formed based on the traditions and paradigms in which we are trained, and emerge and shift in response to new information or the rediscovery of questions and methods.

We suggest that this understanding of the production of knowledge is particularly fitting for population health science. Given population health's concern with readily observed human phenomena, we inevitably come to the discipline with certain preconceived notions, building on particular paradigms emerging within thought collectives. This sociology of science informs the research questions we ask and the way we test hypotheses, which is well substantiated by writing in the medical literature that indicates scientific citations behave in network patterns (Shwed and Bearman 2010, Bayer et al. 2012, Johns et al. 2013) and are informed by value systems and traditions of scholarship.

Thus, we consider population health science principally as a system of science that attempts to gather and judge evidence regarding distributions and burdens of health indicators within and across health systems. Population health science does not aim to uncover one incontrovertible truth that is always the case in all contexts; rather, it is a science that aims to guide our understanding of the complexity of health production across populations, contingent on time, place, and life course influences. This fact makes the field challenging and allows us to draw on insight from a broad range of disciplines, including the more traditional health sciences and also areas as disparate as demography, sociology, and anthropology. As such, population health science is less a collection of methods and more an articulation of values.

Although population health science is perhaps broader in scope and intent than other disciplines, our methods are no less rigorous. To start building the evidence that explicates the chains through which a particular health indicator or disease is caused, our approach in population health science is one we have termed the *causal architecture approach*. Such an approach regards the construction of our theories and hypotheses around disease as a process of placing scaffolding around a building. We construct this scaffolding piece by piece, always drawing the connections among the various parts, looking for parts that work together to build a stronger whole. We elaborate on this approach in Chapters 6 and 7.

3.1 Contrasting Public Health, Population Health Science, and Preventive Medicine

Although in some cases *public health, population health science*, and *preventive medicine* are used interchangeably, we suggest these terms have different meanings, and the nuances of each term should be considered carefully. Population health science is the quantitative underpinning of both public health and preventive medicine, providing practitioners with the evidence from which to base good decisions about implementation, programming, and research agendas specific to various populations of interest. We consider population health science to be the science of understanding the conditions that shape distributions of health in the aggregate, including the mechanisms through which these conditions manifest in the health of individuals within the population. We then endeavor to translate this population health science into policies and programs to improve the health of populations. Preventive medicine, in contrast, is the practice of primary prevention in terms of research programming, policy recommendation, implementation, and clinical practice aimed at preventing the onset of health indicators. Public health is the broader set of efforts—including research programming—aimed at achieving prevention and treatment through large-scale efforts for the population at large. In sum, we see population health science as the beams and bolts that serve as the scaffolding of a broader agenda for both preventive medicine, focused on large-scale efforts through clinical practice, and public health, focused on large-scale efforts through policy, community programming, and implementation. Population health science, then, informs the science that guides our effort to improve public health and prevent disease.

4.0 The First Foundational Principle of Population Health Science

Throughout this book we articulate nine principles of population health science, which are intended to serve as signposts toward a coherent, generative, and forward-looking science. We intend for them to be malleable and debated over time as our field progresses. We articulate in this section the first of these principles.

4.1 What Are Health and Disease at the Population Level?

We are accustomed to thinking of health and disease as happening to us, as individuals, simply because we are all individuals and have all experienced states of health and states of disease. Therefore, when first learning about population health, we tend to think of ourselves as being healthy or sick and applying that thinking to population health scholarship. Today my patient has the flu, hence she is sick. Yesterday she did not, hence she was well. This paradigm—a binary categorization of health and disease—serves us well in our daily lives, both personally and, for those in clinical fields, professionally. When we are sick, we may take a day off from work and may seek help from a physician. This paradigm also serves us well in the practice of medicine, in which doctors are trained to identify illness and to cure it. Medicine, as practiced currently in most countries in the world, is predicated on labeling individuals as sick or healthy. Such labeling is necessary administratively for many purposes, including reimbursement for treatment, consistency in application of treatment, screening guidelines, and decision science. However, such binary classifications rarely reflect the actual distributions of health and the drivers of health in the population.

Population health science requires that we focus on understanding distributions of health rather than their presence or absence. This occasions a different conceptualization of health and disease than the one to which we may be accustomed intuitively. In this book we consider the ways in which health and disease are distributed across populations, and how we as population health scientists are charged with considering the causes of these distributions, rather than the causes of cases. This leads to our first foundational principle (Box 1.1).

There are three central reasons why we consider health as a continuum in population health science. First and foremost, we conceptualize health indicators on continua because, inherently, they are, by and large, continuous in the population. Individuals most often do not simply have or not have a disease or syndrome, and the occurrence, distribution, and severity of symptoms

> **BOX 1.1**
>
> ## First Foundational Principle of Population Health Science
>
> Population health manifests as a continuum.

are not invariant in the population. Thus, a population health science perspective considers the ways in which we can harness this variation in disease severity and progression to understand how distributions of sickness arise and change across populations. Of course, some health indicators are truly binary, the most salient of which, for population health science is death.

Second, although health states within populations often align on a continuum, variations in health states across populations are also inherently continuous, even those health states that are binary (e.g., death). That is, across 100 different cities, we may have substantial variation in the prevalence of lung cancer, and that variation in prevalence travels inherently along a continuum from low to high.

Third, thinking about population health as a continuum, both within a population and between populations, allows us to conceptualize how we can shift the overall health of the population rather than treating or preventing illness on a case-by-case basis. Such a conceptualization is foundational to population health science. We think about "shifting the curve" of population health or focusing on high-risk groups—a concept into which we delve more deeply in Chapter 2. We aim to reduce the number of cases of each poor health outcome and to reduce the mean symptoms, duration, or other factors associated with the health outcome that may exist on these continua.

Fourth, when we conceptualize health as existing on a continuum, it forces us to conceptualize drivers of health as existing similarly on continua, creating opportunity for considering how we may shift the burden of these drivers even slightly and bring about large changes in the health of populations. Factors such as social norms, policies, laws, health behaviors, structural factors, and individual factors are rarely present or absent; they often exist in degrees. By thinking strategically through how we can shift the levels of drivers of population health and continua of symptoms and severity, we can form the most effective, relevant hypothesis tests and subsequent potential inroads to prevention and intervention.

It is worth noting that the notion that health and disease are along a continuum, both at the individual and the population levels, is a concept that is not new to population health science. Perhaps Claude Bernard, French physiologist, prolific author, and early contributor to the science of medicine, said it most eloquently in 1876 in *Lecons sur la chaleur animale* [Lectures on animal heat] (cited by Canguilhem 1978):

> Health and disease are not two essentially different modes as the ancient physicians believed and some practitioners still believe. They should not be made into distinct principles, entities which fight over the living organism and make it the theater of their contest. These are obsolete medical ideas. In reality, between these two modes of being, there are only differences of degree: exaggeration, disproportion, discordance or normal phenomena constitute the diseased state. There is no case where disease would have produced new conditions, a complete change of scene, some new and special product.

4.2 Examples of Population Health as a Continuum

As we think about health indicators as continua, we note that some are conceived easily as such. Blood pressure, CD4 count, body mass index (BMI), or waist circumference, for example, are commonly used metrics for health that are continuous measures. Other health indicators are often conceived of as binary or perhaps ordinal, but a population health science perspective asks us to envision an underlying continuum with respect to the conceptualization of the health outcome. This can be true essentially for any health indicator. For example, infectious diseases are often thought of as present or absent, but most infectious diseases have a wide distribution within and across populations with respect to virulence, number of symptoms, duration, and severity. Furthermore, the prevalence and incidence of infectious diseases vary across populations in ways that are continuous. Even conditions such as Down syndrome, caused by a third copy of chromosome 21, exhibit tremendous variation in the population with respect to ability and capacity, physical limitations, and chronic health sequelae. We consider in Table 1.1 some common health indicators of interest to public health and the ways in which we can conceptualize these health indicators on a continuum. As mentioned, we suggest that only death exists exclusively as a binary state. However, in population health science, we are often more interested in considering death in terms of preventable deaths, and number of years of life lost to premature death, hence providing us with a ready way of considering even death as a continuum.

To illustrate the relation between health continua, binary classifications, and population health, consider Figure 1.1. In Figure 1.1(A), we show a hypothetical distribution of BMI from population A, with a mean value of 23 and a standard deviation of 5, distributed normally. We also show the cutoff of obesity, typically set at 30 kg/m^2. Although in research and public health policy

Table 1.1 Conceptualizing Health on Continua: Examples from Common Health Problems

Health Condition	Binary Conception	Continuum Conception
HIV	Positive diagnosis on blood test	CD4 cell count
Down syndrome	Extra 21st chromosome	Functional ability, cognitive ability, physical limitations
Breast cancer	Positive diagnosis	Tumor stage, characteristics, prognosis
Depression	Meets DSM-V criteria	Number of symptoms, duration of symptoms, comorbidity
Influenza	Laboratory diagnosis	Severity, symptoms, duration, type
Obesity	Body mass index >30	Body mass index value

(American Psychiatric Association 2013).

arenas we discuss the prevalence of obesity, the graph in Figure 1.1(A) illustrates obesity is actually reflective of an underlying continuum of BMIs in the population. Declaring BMI greater than 30 to be the cut point for obesity is based on clinical guidelines and predictive analyses, but it is relatively arbitrary, in that someone with a BMI of 29.9 kg/m^2 and someone with a BMI of 30.1 kg/m^2 are likely at a similar risk for adverse outcomes associated with large body adiposity. In Figure 1.1(B), we add the data from population B. Population B has a mean BMI of 30, with standard deviation 5, and normally distributed values.

Two central themes of note emerge from this example. First, population B has a greater prevalence of obesity than population A, because the mean in population B is much higher than population A. Second, there is some overlap in the distribution of populations A and B such that those with high BMIs in population A have moderate BMIs relative to their respective population means.

As we expand on in Chapters 2 and 3, part of the value in population health thinking is in understanding the powerful effect of population norming on our ability to conceptualize radical changes in population health. If we were only looking within population B, we would not realize that those with moderate BMIs would actually be considered to have a very high BMI if they were to travel to population A.

Thus, considering health as a continuum leads us inexorably to one of the core insights of population health, reframing our question around causation of BMI as: What can we do to shift the entire curve of population B so that the

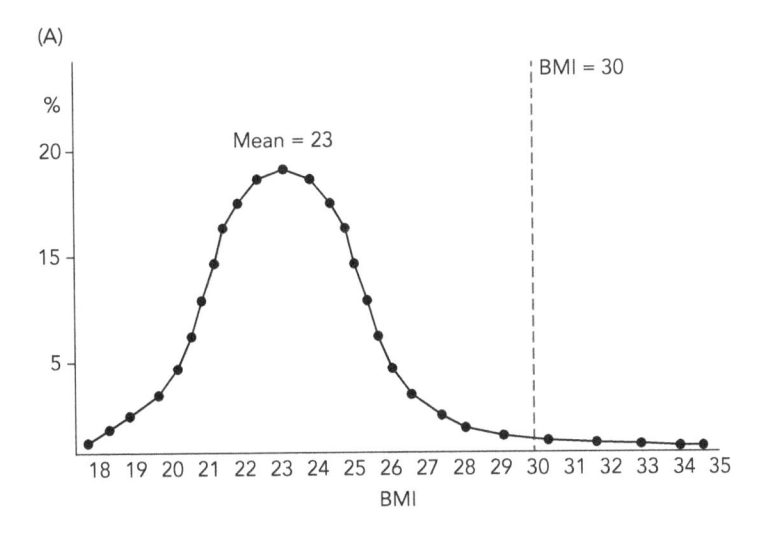

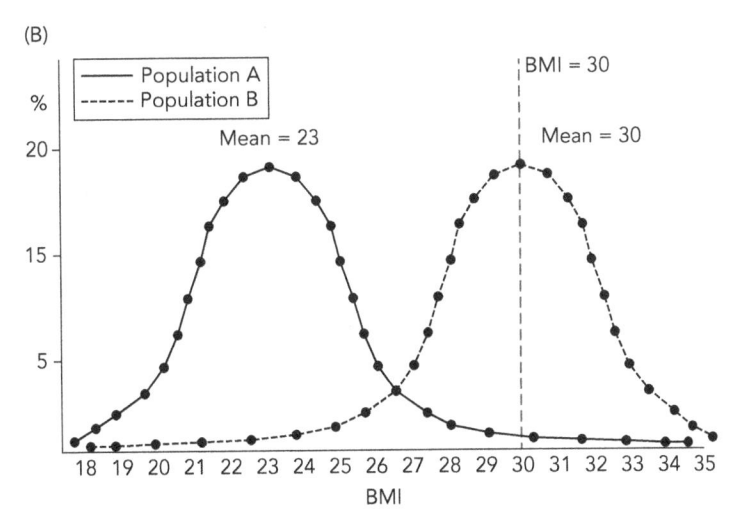

FIGURE 1.1 (A, B) Distribution of body mass index (BMI) in two populations illustrating health as a continuum in the population.

BMIs are more like population A? This question is at the heart of population health science and we return to it again and again throughout this book.

5.0 Organization of the Book

The rest of this book is organized, conceptually, into three parts although we do not demarcate them as such to preserve flow and continuity. First, in Chapters 2 through 6, we discuss the causes of population health, offering both ways to conceive of causes and a framework for thinking about causes to advance population health goals. Second, in Chapters 7 through 9, we discuss how we may weight these causes so that we can identify what matters most toward a consequential population health science. We bring to light the ineluctable role of preventive approaches to any population health science thinking, and how values are critical to our ranking equity and efficiency priorities. Third, in Chapters 10 through 12, we show quantitatively the challenges we face in predicting individual health from population health and how the approaches presented here can inform how we aim to improve the health of populations and promote the equity/efficiency balance that rests at the heart of the field. Chapter 13 concludes with a discussion of the open tensions in population health science with an eye to the future.

6.0 References

American Psychiatric Association. (2013). Diagnostic and statistical manual of mental disorders (5th ed.). Arlington, VA: American Psychiatric Publishing.

Bayer, R., D. M. Johns, and S. Galea. (2012). Salt and public health: contested science and the challenge of evidence-based decision making. *Health Aff (Millwood)* **31**(12): 2738–2746.

Canguilhem, G. (1978). *The normal and the pathological.* Studies in the history of modern science. Dordrecht, Holland: D. Reidel.

Centers for Disease Control and Prevention. (2013). *Centers for Disease Control and Prevention: ten great public health achievements in the 20th century.* Available at: http://www.cdc.gov/about/history/tengpha.htm. Accessed April 22, 2016.

Fleck, L. (1981). *Genesis and development of a scientific fact.* Chicago: University of Chicago Press.

Foucault, M. (1982). The subject and power. *Critical Inquiry* **8**(4): 777–795.

Johns, D. M., R. Bayer, and S. Galea. (2013). Controversial salt report peppered with uncertainty. *Science* **341**(6150): 1063–1064.

Kuhn, T. S. (1962). *The structure of scientific revolutions.* Chicago: University of Chicago Press.

Popper, K. R. (1959). *The logic of scientific discovery.* London: Hutchinson.

Rice, T. (2013). The behavioral economics of health and health care. *Annu Rev Public Health* **34**: 431–447.

Rose, G. A. (1992). *The strategy of preventive medicine.* Oxford: Oxford University Press.

Shwed, U., and P. S. Bearman (2010). The temporal structure of scientific consensus formation. *Am Sociol Rev* **75**(6): 817–840.

Zinszer, K., K. Morrison, A. Anema, M. S. Majumder, and J. S. Brownstein. (2015). The velocity of Ebola spread in parts of West Africa. *Lancet Infect Dis* **15**(9): 1005–1007.

2

Conceptualizing and Evaluating Causes for Population Health Science

POPULATION HEALTH SCIENCE studies the conditions that shape the distributions of health in populations. Central to this study is a concern about understanding the causes of health and disease in populations, why health and disease are distributed differently across populations, and how we can improve the health of populations effectively. It is axiomatic, therefore, that we need to understand the causes of health in populations so we can work to intervene. Causal thinking becomes the exigency of a pragmatic science, a population health science of consequence. This does not mean that causal thinking in population science is straightforward. Nor does it suggest we should focus on isolating the effects of only one cause or the search for singular causes that are the "solution" to complex population health science questions. It does, however, suggest our goal should be to understand the causal architecture of population health so we may intervene effectively to improve the health of populations.

In this chapter we provide a framework for causal thinking for population health science, and articulate and explicate our second foundational principle of population health science: that the causes of population health need consideration separately and apart from the causes of individual health. To get there, though, we first build toward the principle by conceptualizing what a cause is, understanding causes at the individual level, understanding causes at the population level, and understanding their interrelationship.

1.0 What Is a Cause?

The discovery and elucidation of causes is fundamental to any science. In medicine we often want to learn how bodies work so we can understand how and why people get sick, then cure them if they do. In population health science we want to understand the health of populations and the causes of health and disease so we may promote health and prevent disease in populations. As such, central to an introduction to population health science is an explicit consideration of what we mean by *cause* and how we conceptualize causes in population health.

The concept of causation is, on one hand, simple and intuitive and, on the other hand, deeply philosophical and theoretical. Causation is simple and intuitive because we engage in causal inference in our daily lives to survive, thrive, and make decisions. From childhood through adulthood, we judge what is causing certain outcomes so we can avoid those causes, seek them out, or simply understand our world. Infants intuit that crying causes a caregiver to attend to hunger. Adolescents observe that taking a biology class causes knowledge about biology. We also engage, on a daily basis and from an early age, to separate correlation from causation as part of our human experience. As children we learn quickly that the rooster crowing does not cause the sun to come up, for example, despite the correlation between the two. We intuit many facts of the physical and emotional worlds around us without realizing we are engaging in a complicated process of discerning association from causation, and building the causal architecture that governs our behavior and well-being during the day and throughout our lives.

On the other hand, when we think more deeply about how the process of causal inference works, it seems remarkable we are able to engage in these intuitions at all. Causation and causal inference are, in fact, fundamentally philosophical because the process of causation cannot be observed directly; it can only be inferred. Centuries of debate have circled around what it means to say that something is a cause, and how to establish that a causal process has occurred. Certain philosophical traditions or definitions have been established more firmly in particular disciplines and have been passed down through generations of scientists and other scholars, whereas others remain contentious to this day.

At the heart of causal thinking lies a counterfactual paradigm—in other words, a lens on the world that attempts to understand the role a particular cause plays in a controlled universe where we isolate only the particular cause of interest. Counterfactual comparisons are the dominant model for causal thinking in the natural sciences. For example, in physics, if we are trying to understand how a particular force affects the acceleration of a ball, we want to create perfect frictionless conditions for the ball in a vacuum so we can repeat an experiment over and over again in which one cause alone—the applied force—changes and we can then observe what happens to a ball when it is struck. This approach can lead to causal certitude and confidence that one particular factor causes an acceleration of a spherical object of a certain mass. This intuitively pleasing paradigm also guides our thinking about causes in health, even if, as we shall see, it is applied poorly to the production of individual health and is even harder to apply to population health.

Suppose a child falls from a tree and breaks her leg. By observation we infer the fall is what caused the leg to break, which seems like a reasonable assumption. However, to confirm this, we would have to be able to observe that child at the same time in the same place under the condition that she does not fall from the tree to observe that her leg does not break when she does not fall from a tree. This is a metaphysical impossibility bounded by ethics and reality. It is also the complication that bedevils causal thinking in the population health sciences. In the next sections, we first discuss some foundational causal thinking that informs the production of health in individuals and then we build on that scaffolding to think about the production of health in populations.

2.0 Causal Thinking at the Individual Level

Causes of events are those factors necessary for the event to occur when and how it did. Thus, lack of seat belt use would be a cause of death in a car crash if the person would not have died in the crash if the seatbelt was worn. We thus label something a cause of an event if the event would not have occurred without it. We also incorporate timing into the examination of cause, thereby adding to the definition that, for example, the person would not have died when he did without the cause. Death is, unfortunately, inevitable, and there is no cause, or absence of cause, that delays death indefinitely. Thus, a cause of death is something that was necessary for the death to occur when it did; if that particular cause did not occur, the person eventually dies, just at a later date. For example, a smoker might have died 10 years after he did had he not started smoking cigarettes. Abstaining from cigarettes cannot prevent death entirely, but it may contribute to the time that the death occurred. The same logic applies for any health indicator. A cause of cardiac arrest is a factor that contributed to the cardiac arrest occurring when it did;

in the absence of that cause, the cardiac arrest may still have occurred, but at some other time.

When investigating the causes of an event, whether they be states of health or disease, we must consider causes in terms of degree, duration, and intensity. For example, consider the breakup of a romantic relationship. Although there may be some discrete causes we can consider to be contributing factors to the breakup, it also may be the slow accumulation of many causes that together set the stage for the demise of the union. We may not be able to pinpoint one or even a set of specific causes, but we can label the degree, duration, and intensity of the discord over a long period of time as the contributing causes of the relationship breakdown. When the consideration of causes as factors necessary for the event to occur when and how it did is applied to a health context, it is helpful to keep in mind this is a theoretical exercise. We may not be able to pinpoint a single set of causes. Duration and intensity of smoking, for example, may be contributing causes, but we may not be able to specify the exact number of cigarettes that pushed the smoker toward disease. When we consider how and why a person becomes ill, it is helpful to consider causes within the framework we have outlined while acknowledging that a broad and open mind toward the progression of disease allows us to fully contemplate potential population-level causes.

Most events do not have a single cause; they have a cascade of causes that are all needed to be in place for an event to occur. The causes of an event are, thus, all those factors necessary for that event to occur, even if there are many such factors. These causes often accumulate throughout the life course, even from conception or preconception. For example, consider a 55-year-old man who has a heart attack. He is a smoker and has a sedentary lifestyle, and we may ascribe these facts as the causes of the heart attack. This may be correct in the sense that these are the causes most proximal to the event in question. But, we can also take a longer view of the man's life, his parents and their social class, the conditions under which is was born, his education, and other macrolevel factors that may have affected the place and time in which his health behaviors were shaped and, ultimately, created the conditions for the heart attack. A population health perspective requires us to use this broader lens, because our charge as population health scientists is to understand the factors that will prevent many cases of heart attacks—to understand cardiovascular health in the widest sense.

The accumulation of causes through the life course and across levels leads to an understanding that causes are potentially infinite. When we define a cause as a group of factors necessary for an event to occur, and consider causes in the broadest sense, the litany of such causes can quickly become overwhelming. In the case of the girl who falls from the tree and breaks her leg, a necessary factor is climbing the tree; but, this is not the only factor. Other potential causes are poor balance skills, wind velocity, a particular knot in the branch formed by weather patterns during the past decade, poor attentional allocation, insufficient caregiver oversight, choice of neighborhood close to the tree, and myriad other factors. We can even think more broadly than these factors: the girl's age, her choice of clothing that day, her nutritional choices, and her height. All such factors are potentially causes that contributed to the fall. Thus, at the individual level, the causes of an event can be considered in a broad scope, across levels and across time. Yet, as we see in the next section, such thinking may not be helpful in translating causal inference to a population level, when we attempt to discern those causes that create the greatest number of cases. The infinity of cause at the individual level allows us to conceptualize the multiplicity of causal processes through the life course even if our frame of interest—motivated by understanding a small set of potential causes—is often narrow.

Although the list of causes may be infinite, there is also evidence from across disciplines that stochastic processes—chance events—may also explain at least some of the outcomes in both general life and health (Smith 2011). Therefore, prediction of individual events from the set of causes within our frame of interest must acknowledge the futility of determinism. In other words, perhaps part of the reason the girl fell from the tree is back luck. Such stochastic processes may also explain variation in other health indicators as well. In a 2011 review of the role of prediction in population health, Davey Smith noted that experimental studies of marbled crayfish found wide variation in growth and time to mortality, although the crayfish were identical genetically and were bred in the exact same environment (Vogt et al. 2008, Smith 2011). Why one crayfish was big and one was small is likely a series of chance mutations and luck of the draw. Chance, then, plays a role in the production of health at both the individual and the population levels.

In summary, the causes of an event are necessary for that event to occur; accumulate and cascade through the life course in different durations and intensities; may be infinite in scope; and may often involve some degree of stochastic properties. We need not identify all event causes for an individual. This would be futile because of the infinity of causes for many events and because stochastic processes often play a role in event occurrence; thus, we may not be able to determine fully all causes of an event. Why a single individual contracts a disease or is injured whereas another person with the same set of factors does not, involves two general possibilities: (1) there are causes of the event that one person has that the other person does not and (2) even if we were able to identify every cause, stochastic processes could render one person ill and the other person not.

3.0 Conceptualizing Causation at the Population Level

Now that we understand how to conceptualize causes at the individual level, we turn our attention to conceptualizing causes at the population level. Although reasoning why a particular person died or became sick is of great interest to that person and his or her physician, the charge of population health science is to understand the causes of health and disease in populations, why health and disease are distributed differently across populations, and how we can improve the health of populations effectively. These are very different issues than why a particular person became ill.

As mentioned, population health is concerned with the distribution of health and disease across populations. Given the intuitive appeal of thinking about individuals (because, after all, we are all individuals, and are accustomed to thinking of causes in reference to ourselves), it helps to consider the contrast between individual health variation and population health variation. A population health perspective requires us to think beyond individual cases of disease to the distributions of disease and health across populations. Doing so requires a fundamental shift in how we think about causation.

In the first section of this chapter we described how to conceptualize cause for an individual—those factors that necessary for an outcome to occur when and how it did. We then thought about individual variation; within a population, we see that some people are sick and some are not. An important scientific issue—of particular interest to the field of medicine—is to determine why some people are sick and some are not, which we call the process of explaining individual-level variation. However, in population health, we are interested in why some populations have more sickness than others, not why particular individuals within a population are ill. Thus, why some people within the population get sick and some do not is of less interest than why some populations have substantial cases of sickness and some have few. We call such variation—the between-population variation in the incidence and persistence of illness—*population-level variation*.

Conceptualizing and Evaluating Causes for Population Health Science 19

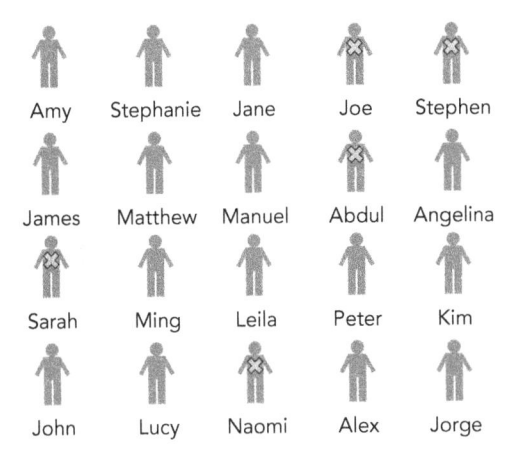

FIGURE 2.1 Conceptualizing causation at the individual level, with 20 students in a classroom.

To illustrate this concept of individual-level variation versus population-level variation, we can think about causation at multiple levels. To understand multiple levels of causation, let us imagine we have a classroom of 20 students, five of whom have asthma: Joe, Sarah, Abdul, Naomi, and Stephen (Figure 2.1).

There is variation in asthma status in this classroom; some students have recurrent asthma attacks and some do not. An important medical question is, for example: Why did Joe develop asthma but Stephanie did not? We may look into their family histories of respiratory problems, home environment, and allergies to determine whether there are any differences between Joe and Stephanie in terms of these potential reasons why Joe developed asthma.

Now let us imagine that we have two classrooms of 20 students each in different schools (Figure 2.2). In classroom 1 (Joe and Stephanie's classroom), five students have asthma, but in classroom 2 there are 10 students with asthma. Instead of asking why Joe developed asthma but Stephanie did not, we ask why there are twice as many cases of asthma in classroom 2 compared with classroom 1.

We can then move beyond looking at classrooms to evaluate the number of cases of asthma in different schools, across districts, across cities, and even across nations. At each level, we are not asking why one child developed asthma whereas another did not (that is, we are not looking at individual-level variation). Instead, we are evaluating why there are more cases of asthma in some places than others (that is, we are looking at population-level variation).

When we evaluate these questions about differences in the burden of asthma across populations with different characteristics (e.g., in different

Classroom 1   Classroom 2

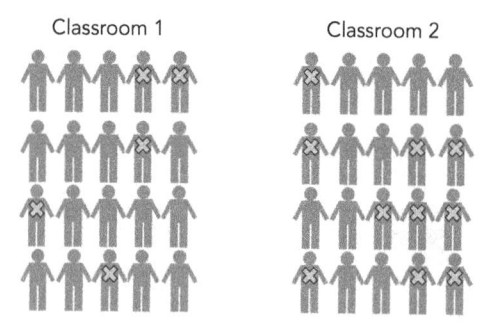

FIGURE 2.2 Conceptualizing causation at the population level by comparing two classrooms.

classrooms, neighborhoods, cities), we are engaging in population health science. At the heart of this science remains the question of cause (i.e., what causes asthma), but the metric on which we evaluate this statement becomes different, with different tools needed to answer causal questions.

Ultimately, the major goal of population health science is to understand what causes health and disease. When we think about "cause" in a population health perspective, however, we shift our frame of thinking from individual-level variation to population-level variation.

The important observation to emerge from this, which is central to population health science, is that the causes of health of populations may well be, and often are, different than the causes of health and disease among individuals within these populations. Returning to the previous example, in our first classroom it may be that Joe, Sarah, Abdul, Naomi, and Stephen were seated in the front row of the class and their asthma attacks were being exacerbated daily by chalk dust from their instructor writing furiously on an old-fashioned chalkboard. Remember that from a formal causal thinking point of view, this might suggest that the same children, in the same classroom, with the same teacher would not have asthma attacks if the teacher used a marker on a whiteboard, hence removing the chalk that causes the asthma attacks.

Therefore, chalk dust is the cause of the asthma attacks. But, when we compare classrooms, there are many more cases of asthma in classroom 2 than there are in classroom 1. This difference is not, plausibly, caused by more chalk dust because, in the similarly configured classrooms, there are the same number of children sitting in the front row in both classes. What could be causing this difference between populations? It may be that classroom 2 is situated at the end of the schoolyard beside a lovely tree that sheds pollen. Therefore, students in classroom 2, all of whom are exposed to a high

BOX 2.1

Second Foundational Principle of Population Health

The causes of differences in health across populations are not necessarily an aggregate of the causes of differences in health within populations.

pollen count, are at a greater risk of an asthma attack than the students in classroom 1. Why, though, do not all students in classroom 2 have asthma, because all are exposed to a high pollen count? This is likely because not all students are equally susceptible to asthma; reactive small-airway disease (asthma) is dependent, to some extent, on genetic vulnerability to the disease. Therefore, the causes of disease rate in population 2 versus population 1 are different than the causes of individual health within either classroom 2 or classroom 1. This observation underlies much of our thinking in population health science and is the foundation of some of our discussion in later chapters. This concept also illustrates the second foundational principle of population health science (Box 2.1).

That is, the causes of variation within a population—why some individuals have the health indicator and some do not—may not be, and often are not, the same factors that cause variation across populations (why some populations have a greater burden of disease than others). We equivocate our principle with "not necessarily" because, in some cases, we may find the causes of individual variation may indeed be the same as the causes of population-level variation. For example, smoking is likely a major determinant of who gets lung cancer and who does not within a population; we would expect, then, that countries with a greater proportion of smokers would have a heavier burden of lung cancer than other countries. In this case, the causes of individual variation may indeed be the same as the causes of population variation. Often, however, we find these causes are indeed separate, both in their conceptualization and in their effects.

4.0 Causal Inference in Population Health Science

Causation cannot be observed; it can only be inferred. Therefore, consistent with the methods of science, the process of establishing causation in population health science requires a careful process of theory building, construction of hypotheses from theory, evaluation of the designs and types of data that inform the hypotheses, and revision of theory based on evidence.

This is done through a reliance on multiple studies, rather than a reliance on single studies, no matter how well designed. In population health science we evaluate the same questions using multiple study designs, each with unique and hopefully nonoverlapping biases, to build an evidence base. We can consider the case for particular causal hypotheses as contributing evidence, ruling on a particular set of exposures or processes through which we are interested in establishing a causal link as the defendants. This is done through the classic scientific method—constructing falsifiable hypothesis tests that advance knowledge, pitting one theory against another, and generating movement forward in our scientific thought processes (Popper 2002).

The process of causal inference in population health science therefore emerges through a series of steps. In population health science, we examine the world in its complexity in an attempt to infer the ways in which health and disease are produced. This is complicated because the world is a complicated place. In some areas of population health science we attempt to abstract this complicated world and answer questions about how single changes in exposures or policies can produce small or large changes in average health. In others, we seek to explain entire systems of health that are interconnected and complicated. Population health science asks us to take a broader view of the processes, means, and strategies through which health is distributed across populations, how much disease is produced by a certain factor or combination of factors, the factors that work together and separately, and the differences between identifying a cause an intervening on that cause.

Acknowledging the uncertainty in our science, however, does not and should not lead us to be afraid of labeling what we are doing as a search for causes. As described earlier in the chapter, all causes are in some way necessary for an event to occur. Several books in the health sciences have tried to differentiate "risk factors" and "causes," under the notion that uncertain causal inference approaches should suggest humility when discussing our associations as potential causes. This leads to the notion that risk factors influence whether an individual becomes sick but do not necessarily cause the outcome to occur. We strongly caution readers against this approach. Anything—any factor, state, characteristic, event, or mechanism necessary for disease to occur in at least some people—can be a cause. We should be fearless about using the term *causation*, because it forces us to pursue causes at all costs, and search for the best data, design, and analysis to answer causal questions.

For example, having a family history of breast cancer increases the risk that a woman will develop breast cancer. However, there are many women who develop cancer who do not have a family history of breast cancer. Does this mean family history is not a cause of breast cancer? That it is merely a "risk factor?" We reject this notion. If there are some women who would not have developed breast cancer if they did not have a family history of breast cancer, then family history is a cause. It should be labeled and treated as such. When we enter the murky world of separating risk factors from the so-called true causes, we move away from opening ourselves up to the plethora of intervention opportunities that may have the greatest impact on population health. The oft-used aphorism "correlation is not causation"—although important as we endeavor always to be critical of our work—can sometimes force us to shy away from truly engaging in a thought process about the causal architecture that we theorize can underlie the associations that we are observing. We ward readers away from such timidity.

5.0   References

Popper, K. (2002). *The logic of scientific discovery*. London: Routledge Classics.

Smith, G. D. (2011). Epidemiology, epigenetics and the 'Gloomy Prospect': embracing randomness in population health research and practice. *Int J Epidemiol* 40(3): 537–562.

Vogt, G., M. Huber, M. Thiemann, G. van den Boogaart, O. J. Schmitz, and C. D. Schubart. (2008). Production of different phenotypes from the same genotype in the same environment by developmental variation. *J Exp Biol* 211(Pt 4): 510–523.

3

The Causes of Cases Versus Causes of Incidence

IN THE PREVIOUS two chapters we introduced two foundational population health principles: (1) population health manifests on a continuum and (2) the causes of population health are often distinct from the causes of individual cases within a population. With this background in place, in this chapter we build on these concepts and explore in greater depth the idea that population-level causes may be different than individual-level causes. To do so we divided this chapter in into three parts: first, we use as our foundation the work of Geoffrey Rose to illustrate the concept of individual-level versus population-level causes. This includes the concept of *ubiquitous causes*, to which we return in Chapter 5. Second, we expand on the principles described by Rose by including two quantitative examples that illustrate how and when individual-level causes and population-level causes differ. Third, we discuss how prevention strategies can make substantial differences in population health, by building on Rose's work and discussing the difference between approaches that focus on high-risk individuals and approaches that aim to shift the population health curve.

1.0 Causes of Cases Within Populations and Causes of Incidence Across Populations

Causation is foundational to population health science. We need to know what causes disease so we can develop and test approaches that reduce disease burden in populations. In some ways this is intuitive. We understand health and disease at the individual level, in that a patient is sick or healthy. However, a population health perspective requires us not to think about individuals with disease, but rather populations with disease.

Geoffrey Rose articulated this perspective best and foundationally as the field of population health science was starting to take shape (Rose 1985, Rose et al. 2008). He posed the issue of causation in a population health perspective by considering the distribution of blood pressure in two populations: London civil servants and Kenyan nomads. We can think of each of these two populations as having a distribution with respect to blood pressure.

Consider Figure 3.1, based on the example provided in Rose (1985) in which each circle represents a different hypothetical London civil servant (note that our figure is a teaching example only and is not based on actual data). We chart the systolic blood pressures of each civil servant along an axis and align each person with the same blood pressure in a column. We see there are some individuals with very low blood pressure and some individuals with very high blood pressure, but there are only a few people at these extremes. Most are near the center of the graph, with a systolic blood pressure of about 135 mmHg. Thus, within this population we have a distribution of blood pressures, from low to high. This also represents the population base on which we typically ask questions concerning the production of health. Therefore, within this population, we can ask why some people have very low systolic blood pressure whereas others have very high blood pressure, and we might find that what causes this variation within the civil servants may be, in part, a result of genetic differences, diet, and exercise, among other factors.

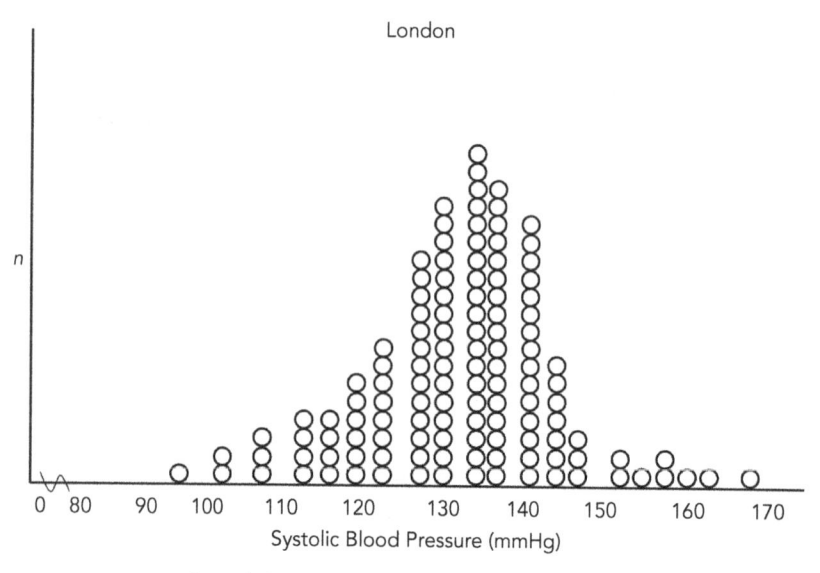

FIGURE 3.1 Hypothetical data on the systolic blood pressure of London civil servants.

Kenya

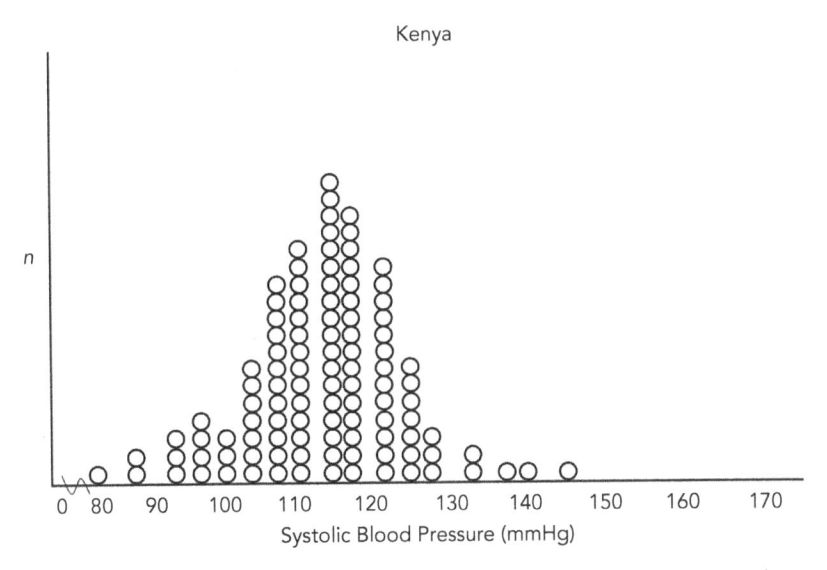

FIGURE 3.2 Hypothetical data on the systolic blood pressure of Kenyan nomads.

Now, however, we provide the same type of data—a circle for each person—for a population of Kenyan nomads (Figure 3.2). We see the same bell-shaped curve, with some very low and some very high values, but most people cluster toward the middle. Again, we might consider the factors that, among Kenyan nomads, make some people have higher blood pressure and some people have lower. The reality is likely a combination of genetic differences, diet, and exercise.

The causal question we now ask—Why do some people have a higher blood pressure than others?—likely contains answers within both the London and Kenyan populations that can help us identify individuals who are at risk for high blood pressure and whose high blood pressure we may therefore try to control.

However, this approach is missing a very important observation. The entire population, or, the population "curve" of blood pressure, is, on average, much less in the Kenyan nomads than in the London civil servants. Those who would be considered as having very high blood pressure in the nomad group are at the same blood pressure considered average for the London group. These data, then, reveal a question hidden by the study of any single population alone: why does the blood pressure curve lie where it does? Why do we have a higher mean, and higher distribution of blood pressure, among London civil servants than we do among Kenyan nomads? And, critically, the reasons why Kenyan nomads have, on average, lower blood pressure compared with London civil servants may be very different than the reasons why some London civil servants have higher blood pressure than others.

Rose termed this the difference between understanding "sick individuals and sick populations." That is, the distributions of sickness across populations may have causes that are unique from the causes of individual differences within populations. The corollary to this, of course, is that acting to improve the health of populations does not necessarily mean we are improving the lives of particular individuals within those populations.

The central implication of the perspective advanced by Rose, and embedded in this principle, is that the causes of cases may be distinct from the causes of incidence, and when we consider why only some people have the disease and some do not by looking within a population, we may be missing critical causes of the disease itself. There are clearly any number of differences that characterize the living conditions of London civil servants and Kenyan nomads. The former live in a densely populated urban environment whereas the latter may predominately reside on grassy plains. Civil servants have rigid daily routines whereas Kenyan nomads' lives are based on farm and livestock upkeep. Therefore, an approach that aims to understand what causes high blood pressure might tell us that, within a population, sedentary persons have higher blood pressure, which might have us looking to identify sedentary persons so we may reduce their risk of high blood pressure. However, would it not be much more effective if we could understand the characteristic of the population—perhaps the feature of the urban environment—that results in all civil servants having higher blood pressure than the nomads? If we could do that, we would then be able to "shift" the population curve, improving the health of an entire population, rather than that of individuals, one at a time.

The difference between causes of cases and causes of incidence can also be illustrated simply and mathematically. Consider the following example. Suppose we are interested in preventing a disease called *populosis* and, unbeknown to us, populosis has two causes: genetic vulnerability and environmental exposure. In our population there is variance in genetic composition—meaning, some individuals are at genetic risk for populosis and some are not; however, everyone is exposed to the same environment. Thus, there is no variance in environment. Because there is only one other cause of populosis, then within our population, the reason that some people have populosis is based on their genetic vulnerability only. Why is this a problem? Because if we are able to discern that environmental exposure is causing disease, we could potentially prevent the environmental exposure and reduce disease substantially. However, we need to compare environments across populations to observe the effect of the environment on populosis. This is when comparing populations and aspiring to understand the cause of incidence in populations comes into play.

We are presenting here a particular case of population causation—namely, cases when a cause of disease is ubiquitous in a population. In this case we often cannot "see" the effect of that cause. We are only able to infer the effect of that cause by determining the overall burden of disease is higher in one population than another. But, within a population, ubiquitous causes are often silent. Importantly, of course, just because we cannot see the cause in our data does not mean the cause is not creating cases.

We all understand why we may want to learn the causes of cases. At the core, we want to understand what causes disease in ourselves or in a patient. However, in the field of population health science, we often want to understand the broader ways in which we can prevent disease, in which we can "shift the curve" of population health. To do so, we need to completely understand the factors that cause disease. By taking a population health approach, we have to broadly conceptualize the potential drivers of health distributions (rather than cases) across populations and find ways to examine variance in those causes so we can identify the causes of population health, even if they are ubiquitous.

2.0 Quantitative Examples of Population Health Causation

Thus far we have explained that the factors that cause variation in health status within a population may be different than the factors that cause variation in health status across populations. Rose (1985) demonstrated this principle elegantly more than 20 years ago with the example of blood pressure among London civil servants and Kenyan nomads, leading to the idea that we could shift the curve of population health by focusing on those causes that are ubiquitous within a population and variant across populations. In this section we provide two quantitative examples to numerically illustrate the implications that within-population differences may have for health compared with between-population differences. In particular, we illustrate cases when the between-population and within-population causes are different, but are, in the first case, independent and, in the second case, dependent on one another.

2.1 Example 1: When Between-Population Causes and Within-Population Causes Are Distinct and Independent: High Cholesterol

In this example, we show results for two populations in which the causes of variation within the population are the same and yet the rate of the outcome differs across the populations.

We have two hypothetical populations, which we term population Chadwick and population Farr. We are interested in the determinants of low-density lipoprotein (LDL) cholesterol in each of these populations. For the sake of simplicity, there are two causes of LDL cholesterol: chronic poverty conditions in childhood and eating potato chips in adulthood. We start an investigation to determine the association between eating chips and LDL cholesterol in each population, with data presented in Figure 3.3.

As indicated in Figure 3.3, population Chadwick has a mean LDL cholesterol of 170 mg/dL with a standard deviation of 33.3 mg/dL. Using a standard cutoff of "high" LDL cholesterol of 190 mg/dL, we estimate the total number of cases of high LDL cholesterol among those who eat potato chips versus those who do not eat potato chips. Our estimates for population Chadwick are shown in Table 3.1, and below we estimate the risk difference in high LDL cholesterol between those who eat potato chips and those who do not.

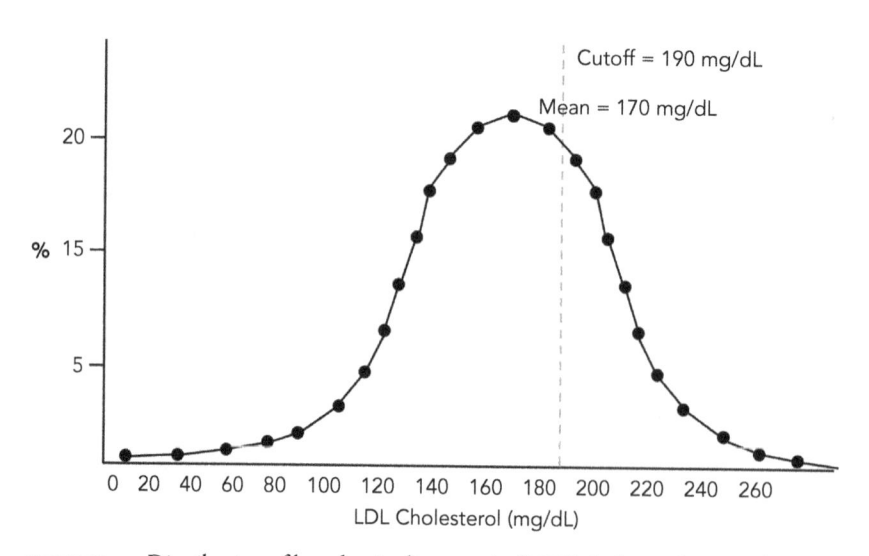

FIGURE 3.3 Distribution of low-density lipoprotein (LDL) cholesterol in population Chadwick.

Table 3.1 The Relation between Potato Chip Eating and Cholesterol in Population Chadwick

	High LDL Cholesterol, n	Low LDL Cholesterol, n	Total, n
Chip eater	150	350	500
Not a chip eater	125	375	500
Total	275	725	1000

$$\text{Risk difference} = \left(\frac{150}{500}\right) - \left(\frac{125}{500}\right) = 0.05$$

Based on the answer from the previous equation, there are five additional cases of high LDL cholesterol for every 100 additional chip eaters.

As shown in Figure 3.4, population Farr has a mean LDL cholesterol of 140 mg/dL with a standard deviation of 35.7 mg/dL.

Using the same cutoff as in population Chadwick, we now estimate the total number of cases of high LDL cholesterol among those who eat chips versus those who do not. Our estimates for population Farr are given in Table 3.2, and the risk difference is provided below.

$$\text{Risk difference} = \left(\frac{50}{500}\right) - \left(\frac{25}{500}\right) = 0.05$$

Based on the answer from the previous equation, in population Farr, as in population Chadwick, there are five additional cases of high LDL cholesterol for every 100 additional chip eaters.

To summarize, we obtain the same risk difference in population Chadwick and population Farr for the association between chip eating and high LDL cholesterol, and both populations have the same prevalence of chip eating. But, the overall risk of high LDL cholesterol is the difference between the two populations. In population Chadwick, 27.5% of the population has high LDL cholesterol compared with 7.5% of the population in population Farr.

Thus, within the population, potato chip eating is a risk factor for high LDL cholesterol, and the same number of excess cases of high LDL cholesterol resulting from chip eating are observed in both populations. Yet, population Chadwick has a much greater risk of high LDL cholesterol. Why is this the case?

Suppose we later discover that the adults in population Chadwick spent their childhood in poverty whereas those in population Farr did not.

32 POPULATION HEALTH SCIENCE

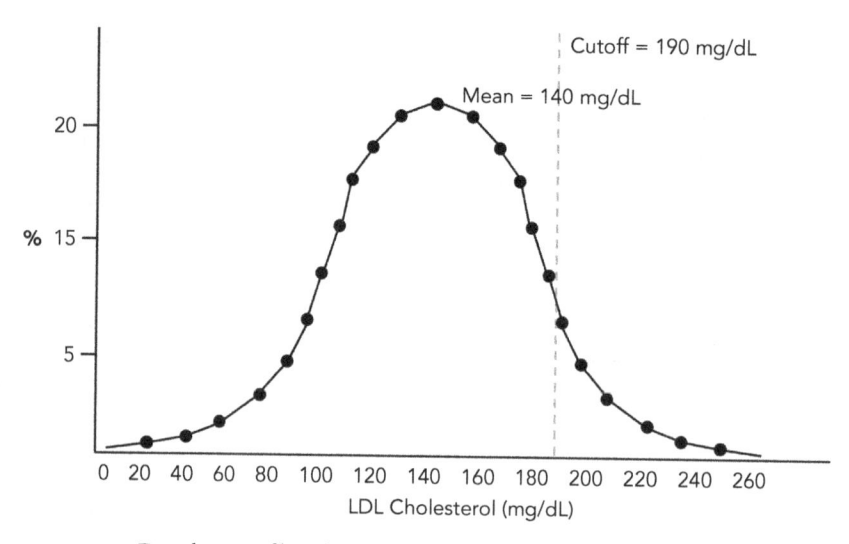

FIGURE 3.4 Distribution of low-density lipoprotein (LDL) cholesterol in population Farr.

If chronic childhood poverty is also a cause of high LDL cholesterol, then the between-population differences in the overall risk of high LDL cholesterol can be explained, at least in part, by childhood poverty, although the differences within each population can be explained by chip eating.

Let us reorganize the data with the "exposure" being childhood poverty, assuming all those in population Chadwick are exposed and all those in population Farr are not exposed to childhood poverty. We disregard who is a chip eater and who is not. Our data are shown in Table 3.3, and the risk difference for high LDL cholesterol between those exposed to childhood poverty versus those not exposed is shown below.

$$\text{Risk difference} = \left(\frac{275}{1000}\right) - \left(\frac{75}{1000}\right) = 0.20$$

Table 3.2 The Relation between Potato Chip Eating and Cholesterol in Population Farr

	High LDL Cholesterol, n	Low LDL Cholesterol, n	Total, n
Chip eater	50	450	500
Not a chip eater	25	475	500
Total	75	925	1000

LDL, low-density lipoprotein.

Table 3.3 The Relation between Childhood Poverty and Cholesterol in Both the Chadwick (All Exposed to Childhood Poverty) and Farr (All Unexposed to Childhood Poverty) Populations

	High LDL Cholesterol, n	Low LDL Cholesterol, n	Total, n
Childhood poverty	275	725	1000
No childhood poverty	75	925	1000
Total	350	1650	2000

LDL, low-density lipoprotein.

Thus, when we combine populations and examine the factor that caused the difference in the overall risk of high LDL cholesterol between populations (childhood poverty), we see there is an excess of 20 cases of high LDL cholesterol for every 100 adults exposed to childhood poverty across these populations. Assuming these are causal effects, we would prevent more LDL cholesterol by preventing childhood poverty than by preventing people from eating chips, although eating chips is a cause of high LDL cholesterol.

This is not to say that healthy eating should not also be encouraged, but a population health science perspective requires us to examine the broad range of factors across levels of organization and across populations to determine the most ubiquitous and harmful causes of disease overall, thereby allowing us to focus on prevention and intervention that have the most meaningful impact on population health. In this example, although encouraging people to eat a healthy diet is an important public health goal for many different reasons, we can see that childhood poverty is responsible for more overall cases and might, as such, be an important focus of public health concern.

2.2 Example 2: When Between-Population Causes and Within-Population Causes Are Distinct and Dependent: Depressive Symptoms

In our second example, we show results for two populations in which an exposure is associated with a health indicator, but the magnitude of the association differs across populations as a result of differences in the prevalence of interacting causes.

Major depressive disorder is a condition characterized by persistent and disabling feelings of sadness, worthlessness, anhedonia, as well as sleep and appetite disturbance, psychomotor agitation, and thoughts of suicide. Depression is one of the leading causes of disability worldwide and is one of the most prevalent medical conditions in many countries, including the United States (Ferrari et al. 2013). Known risk factors for depression include a family history of the disorder or other psychiatric conditions, a childhood history of adversity or abuse, loss of a loved one and other personally traumatic experiences, alcohol and other substance use, and socially patterned factors likely linked to structural population health causes such as race/ethnicity, sex, and geographic location.

For our example, we again assume two hypothetical populations and, for the sake of simplicity, generate a very simple causal structure for depression incidence. In this example, we assume alcohol use is a cause of depression and that the effect of alcohol use on depression is stronger among those of younger age than those of older age. All other causes of depression are assumed to be independent of age and alcohol use and are distributed similarly across the two populations. We start an investigation to determine the association between alcohol use and depression incidence in each of our two hypothetical populations.

We measure depression with a scale that counts the number of symptoms reported by members of the population, normalized to a distribution from 0 to 100. As seen in Figure 3.5, population Chadwick has a mean of 40 depressive symptoms with a standard deviation of 15.4. We assume for this example that depressive symptoms are distributed normally. We dichotomize the depression symptoms so that anyone with more than 60 has "probable depression," and estimate the total number of cases of probable depression among those

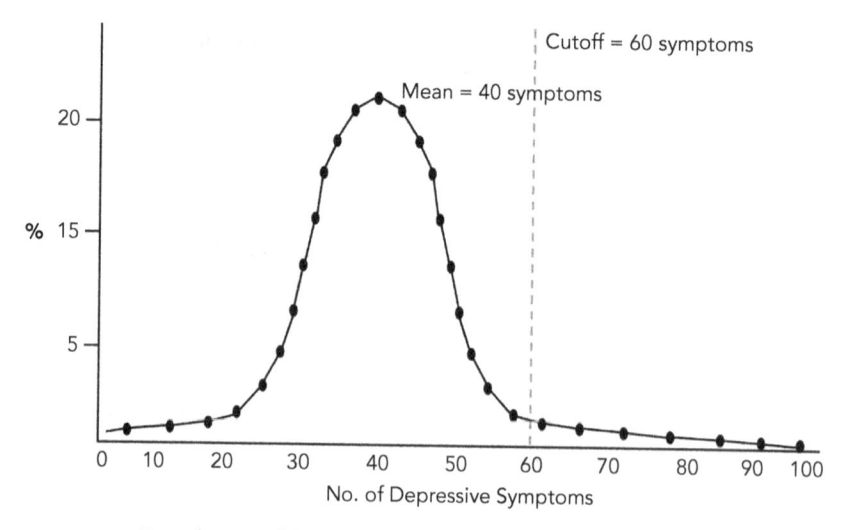

FIGURE 3.5 Distribution of depressive symptoms in Chadwick.

Table 3.4 Probable Depression among Those Who Are Chronic Heavy Alcohol Consumers and among Those Who Are Not in Population Chadwick

	Probable Depression, n	No Probable Depression, n	Total, n
Chronic heavy alcohol consumption	75	425	500
No chronic heavy alcohol consumption	25	475	500
Total	100	900	1000

who are chronic heavy alcohol consumers versus those who are not. Our estimates for population Chadwick are presented in Table 3.4, with the risk difference comparing heavy chronic alcohol consumers versus others shown below.

$$\text{Risk difference} = \left(\frac{75}{500}\right) - \left(\frac{25}{500}\right) = 0.10$$

According to our calculations, there are 10 additional cases of probable depression for every 100 additional chronic heavy alcohol consumers.

Population Farr has 60 mean depression symptoms with a standard deviation of 15.4 (Figure 3.6). Using the same cutoff as in Chadwick, we now estimate the total number of cases of probable depression among those who are chronic heavy alcohol consumers versus those who are not. Our estimates for Farr are shown in Table 3.5, and again, the risk difference comparing heavy chronic alcohol consumers versus others shown below.

$$\text{Risk difference} = \left(\frac{250}{500}\right) - \left(\frac{135}{500}\right) = 0.23$$

The previous equation indicates there are 23 additional cases of probable depression for every 100 additional chronic heavy alcohol consumers.

Now, in contrast to example 1, we see that not only does population Farr have more probable depression than population Chadwick, but the magnitude of the association between alcohol consumption and depression is greater in population Farr than in population Chadwick. Suppose, then, that the age distributions of the two populations differ and there are more young

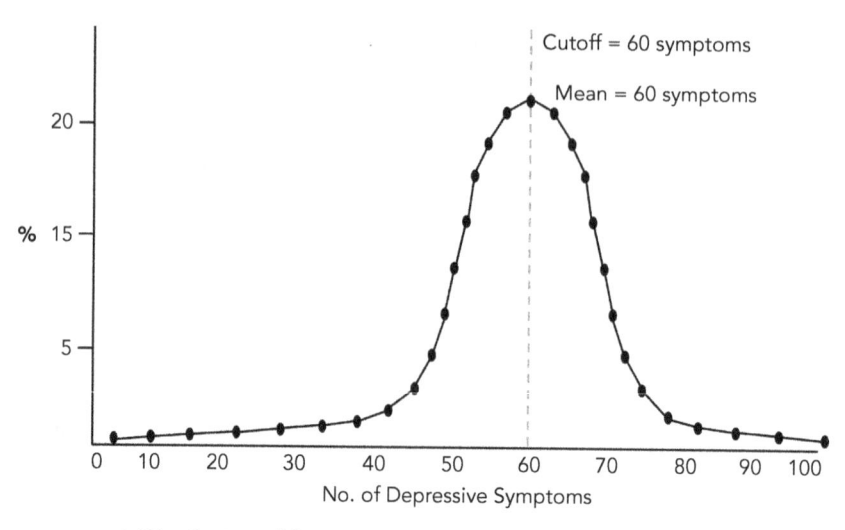

FIGURE 3.6 Distribution of depressive symptoms in Farr.

people in population Farr than in population Chadwick. If the effects of alcohol consumption on depression were greater among younger individuals than older persons, we would expect not only more cases, but also more cases resulting from the effects of chronic alcohol consumption in population Farr compared with population Chadwick.

Thus, in example 2, if we want reduce probable depression by focusing on alcohol consumption, we will have a greater impact on population distributions of depressive symptoms by focusing on the population with a younger age distribution. This is, in many ways, intuitive; we want to focus on populations at greater risk for developing the outcome if our exposure of interest is especially pernicious among those at greater risk. This idea has certainly been a foundation of screening programs for many years; we screen high-risk populations because the

Table 3.5 Probable Depression among Those Who Are Chronic Heavy Alcohol Consumers and among Those Who Are Not in Population Farr

	Probable Depression, n	No Probable Depression, n	Total, n
Chronic heavy alcohol consumption	250	250	500
No chronic heavy alcohol consumption	135	365	500
Total	385	615	1000

predictive value of a positive screening test increases as the prevalence of the disease increases. So, too, can we apply these principles to population health. When exposures interact with other factors, our exposures have increased predictive validity (and thus magnitude of association) when we examine them in populations at greater baseline risk, such as the young population in our example.

In example 1, the causes of variation within the population are different than the causes of variation across populations, but those causes are independent of each other. In example 2, the causes of variation within the population are different than the causes of variation across populations, and these causes are not independent of each other. In both examples, understanding how the distributions of causes differ across populations is critical in understanding population health. This again illustrates population health science foundational principle 2 (the causes of differences in population health are not necessarily an aggregate of the causes of differences in individual health), first introduced in Chapter 2. However, we must also be keenly aware of how causes within and across populations relate to each other. If the effect of one cause moderates the effect of another cause, then the associations differ within populations as well as across populations. This indicates that population health is often caused by a complex causal architecture in which estimating risk ratios and other magnitudes of association requires a critical eye toward how causes function not only in isolation, but also in conjunction with other causes.

3.0 Prevention Strategies for Population Health

Thus far we have demonstrated that causes of variation within the population and causes of variation between populations may be distinct. We have also demonstrated that when causes interact, a change in the prevalence of one cause across populations may have a substantial impact on the number of cases produced by the other cause. Yet, the main goal of identifying these causes within and across populations is, ultimately, to keep people and populations healthy.

This population paradigm suggests two dominant frameworks that can be used to harness the information we have about causes in populations to identify how to improve health. Each has costs and benefits that should be weighed and considered. We articulate each strategy in the following sections.

3.1 Focusing on High-Risk Groups

In population health science we are interested in identifying groups who are at high risk of developing disease. We do this by examining data for the characteristics of persons who develop disease compared with the characteristics of persons who do not. We identify those characteristics, traits, or comorbidities that predict the occurrence of disease to more completely characterize those who will and will not develop an illness. For example, persons at greater risk for the development of cardiovascular disease are men, those who smoke, those who consume high amounts of saturated fat, and those with greater adiposity and a sedentary lifestyle. In contrast, those at greater risk for ovarian cancer include women who are nulliparous, who use certain fertility-promoting medications, and who have a family history of reproductive cancers. We identify such factors so we can understand the etiology of these health indicators and, importantly, so that we may potentially design intervention and prevention programs that target such groups.

A "high-risk strategy" is one in which we address specifically these groups at greater risk for health indicators by using screening, targeted health messaging, and other programs that consider the characteristics of individuals to stratify who receives an intervention and who does not. Examples of high-risk strategies can be seen throughout clinical medicine and public health. Women with a family history of breast cancer, for example, are advised to undergo routine mammography screening earlier than women without such a history. The logic of such a guideline is that by focusing on those at greater risk than others, we can direct resources to those who are most likely to need those resources, such as early mammography screening. The incidence of breast cancer among women in their 40s without a family history of breast cancer is low, indicating the cost of screening them is not an effective public health strategy, and that screening can do more harm than good if invasive procedures are introduced among false-positive cases. Public health high-risk strategies include providing free condoms to adolescents visiting a health clinic, treating individuals with blood pressure greater than a certain level with hypertensive medication or those with cholesterol greater than a certain level with statins, or additional genetic and prenatal testing for pregnant women of advanced age.

Although risk factors for disease are often assessed empirically at a population level, the implementation of high-risk screening and prevention strategies is most often an individualized approach facilitated within a medical care setting. That is, individuals present for care and physicians or other health professionals assess their risk factors and make recommendations based on these risk factors. For some health indicators, this may be the most cost-effective approach to reducing the population burden of disease, based on the distribution of those risk factors in the population, their functional form, the amenability of the risk factors to intervention, and the probability that intervention will reduce population burden of disease.

3.2 Focusing on the Population

An alternative, or adjunct, approach to focusing on high-risk groups is to focus on the population as a whole. This approach advocates a theoretical model of *shifting the curve*, as it is often termed. That is, rather than focus on groups and high risk of disease and attempting to prevent disease among them, we attempt to change the overall mean, shifting the value incrementally for each individual. For example, if we are interested in reducing alcohol-related harm, a high-risk approach is to prevent or reduce alcohol consumption among those who drink the most, but not intervening to reduce alcohol consumption among moderate drinkers. Alternatively, a population approach is to develop a program that reduces alcohol consumption by one or several drinks per week for the whole population of drinkers.

Such an approach is likely to be most effective under several conditions. First, given that shifting the curve of population health typically requires large-scale changes to public health practice and policy, political and social will needs to be available to engage in large-scale efforts toward population change. Second, at a practical level, a population approach is most applicable when the exposures of interest have a dose–response or monotonic relationship with the outcome. That is, when there is no clear threshold on which to label a group as high risk, an approach that focuses on shifting the entirety of the distribution may produce a better population-level outcome.

As we have described throughout this chapter, health indicators and their risk factors of interest are often arrayed on a continuum in a population. Understanding this foundational principle is central to understanding population health. When we acknowledge that health is arrayed on a continuum, we can see the benefit of shifting the whole curve upward or downward as opposed to truncating the distribution only at one end by focusing on high-risk groups.

There are many examples of population approaches to public health in the literature. Consider motor vehicle crash fatality in which both high-risk and population approaches have combined to reduce fatalities dramatically during the 20th century in the United States (Centers for Disease Control and Prevention 1999). Systematic population approaches have been taken, including improving vehicle safety, enforcing policies and laws to require seat belt use, and creating infrastructure changes to improve road conditions and signage. These improvements were not targeted at particular individuals at high risk for a crash; they are population-wide in scope and implementation. At the same time, however, efforts have been made to reduce alcohol-impaired driving through the passage and enforcement of laws and the creation public health campaigns to change social norms regarding drinking and driving. We could consider this a high-risk approach because those who drive while intoxicated are a very high-risk group for causing injury to self and others. Other examples of community-based population approaches include the North Karelia project in Finland, which focused on improving cardiovascular disease risk for the whole population rather than any particular groups (Puska et al. 1983), and other population-wide public health programming including vaccination, water fluoridation, and food fortification.

To summarize, when we consider intervention and prevention on health indicators in the population, there are two main approaches: focus on reducing risk among high-risk individuals and focus on reducing risk for the entire population. These approaches are summarized in Figure 3.7.

3.3 Comparing High-Risk Versus Population Approaches

A high-risk approach is often at odds with the broad scope population health approaches we highlight and advocate in this text. High-risk strategies often place the burden of prevention at the hands clinical care systems working with patients one-on-one, rather than placing a focus at the population level on strategies that can shift the entire population burden of disease. Although a focus on the individual level can be transformative (e.g., screening and prevention based on specific genetic profiles when such profiles are associated strongly with disease), in other ways, such as those that focus on behavioral factors including diet, substance use, and lifestyle, these approaches can ignore the broader cultural and social landscape that shapes the emergence of these behaviors. A population approach allows us the possibility of imagining interventions that are broad in scope and in concept; in contrast, a high-risk approach often limits our ability truly to transform public health because the focus is often on individual identification of cases and individual behavior chance. Prevention becomes a real possibility when we start thinking about populations and shifting the curve of health for all members of the population regardless of underlying risk. We expand further on this point, providing quantitative examples of high-risk and prevention approaches, in Chapter 12.

Furthermore, unless the factors that place individuals at high risk are strongly associated with the disease, identification of individuals based on these factors is unlikely to affect population health robustly. For example, an odds ratio of 3.0 (that is, those with the risk factor have three times the odds of developing the disease compared with those who do not) is considered a strong relation in most epidemiological studies. Simulation analyses

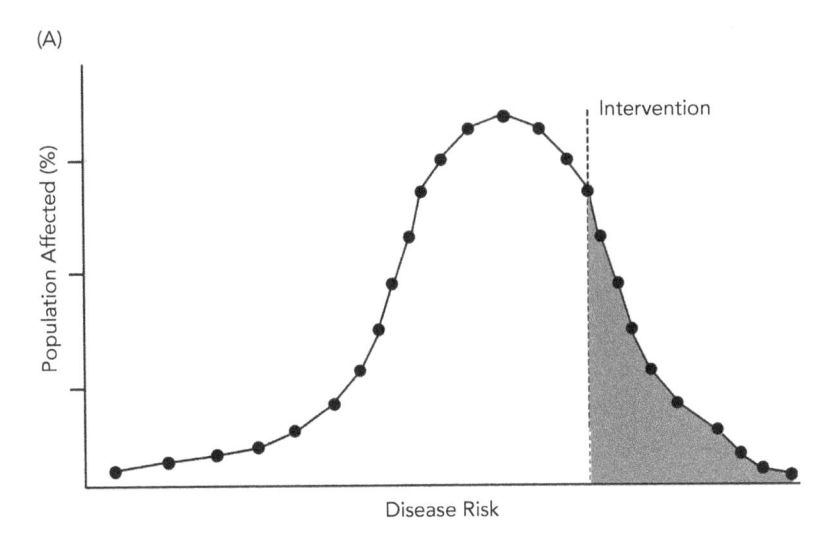

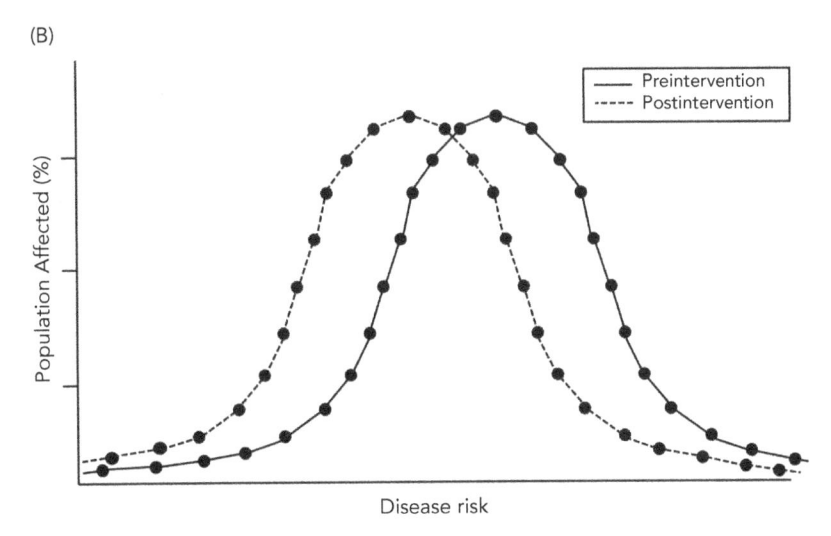

FIGURE 3.7 (A, B) High-risk (A) and population (B) approaches to disease prevention.

have demonstrated, however, that even an odds ratio of 3.0 has little predictive power for determining which individuals actually develop the disease or not. Odds ratios on the order of magnitude of 70.0, 80.0, or more are most predictive (Pepe et al. 2004) and few associations that we observe in human populations have such strong predictive power.

As an example, suppose we are evaluating potential ways to reduce cardiovascular disease, in a world of finite resources. We can either treat those with high blood pressure or cholesterol with medication, or we can invest in a national effort aimed at nutritious school lunch programs for preschoolers through students in grade 6. We know that antihypertensive medications and statins work to lower blood pressure and cholesterol, and will likely prevent at least some heart disease from occurring in those who take the medication as prescribed. But the approach is individualized. To be treated successfully, individuals must have sufficient resources to see a physician, and the health literacy to understand instructions, take prescribed medications, and adhere to protocols. On the other hand, we know the trajectory of obesity, which is related to heart disease in adulthood, begins early in life and can be difficult to change after onset has begun. If we could prevent obesity and encourage a nutritious diet at a very young age, we may prevent more cases of heart disease than with an individualized approach in adulthood, but these wins would not be realized for decades. Thus, the former has an immediate but potentially limited impact whereas the latter has a broader but delayed impact.

The decision to engage with a high-risk approach or a population approach depends, on some degree, on the public's comfort level with what Rose terms *the prevention paradox*: "a preventive measure that brings large benefits to the community offers little to each participating individual" (Rose 1981, p. 1847). Put succinctly, a population approach to disease prevention requires that many people in the population modify some aspect of health-related behavior or habits, but the preventive intervention will never benefit most of those individuals, because most people will not die or become ill in any case from the health outcome. If we convince everyone in the population to reduce alcohol consumption per day by one drink, we may see a population benefit that is much greater than if we focused only on convincing the very heavy drinkers to quit. But, for that benefit, many individuals who never would develop any problems related to their alcohol use would have had to curtail their nightly cocktail. This example informs our third foundational principle of population health (Box 3.1). This principle underlies some of the core challenges faced by population health science in conveying its utility even as

---

BOX 3.1

Third Foundational Principle of Population Health Science

Large benefits to population health may not improve the lives of all individuals.

some individuals do not necessarily realize benefits from population health approaches.

The perils of the prevention paradox, this tradeoff between what is good for the individual and what is good for the population, has been playing out in the front pages of newspapers as parents opt out of vaccinating their children. At an individual level, parents can argue they may take preventive measures with their children, such as hand washing and quarantine during illness, and they do not want to risk an adverse vaccine-related event. The potential consequence of this of course is the emergence of measles and other epidemics of vaccine-preventable illness in communities in the United States and elsewhere.

Population health interventions face other challenges as well. Decisions regarding population versus high-risk approaches must take into account the potential risks of the approach for individuals at low probability of the outcome. Any population approach often involves exposing a large portion of individuals to factors we think are going to improve the overall population's health (or conversely, removing an exposure from individuals). The size and scale of such programs imposes a burden on population health scientists for making an unequivocal case that the benefit from the population intervention well outweighs the benefits of a focus on high-risk groups, mitigating potential unanticipated risk.

4.0 Summary

In summary, population health science is the study of the conditions that shape distributions of health in populations. Therefore, population health science rests on a robust understanding of populations. Population causes are often different than the sum of individual causes. Populations represent the interaction of individuals with their context, and are influenced by causes at multiple levels. The work of Geoffrey Rose was among the first to illustrate these concepts. Extending the work of Rose leads us to an understanding of the centrality of preventive approaches to the promotion of population health through a focus on the causes of population health, shifting the population curve of health.

5.0 References

Centers for Disease Control and Prevention. (1999). Motor-vehicle safety: a 20th century public health achievement. *MMWR Morb Mortal Wkly Rep* **48**(18): 369–374.

Ferrari, A. J., F. J. Charlson, R. E. Norman, S. B. Patten, G. Freedman, C. J. Murray, T. Vos, and H. A. Whiteford. (2013). Burden of depressive disorders by country, sex, age, and year: findings from the global burden of disease study 2010. *PLoS Med* **10**(11): e1001547.

Pepe, M. S., H. Janes, G. Longton, W. Leisenring, and P. Newcomb. (2004). Limitations of the odds ratio in gauging the performance of a diagnostic, prognostic, or screening marker. *Am J Epidemiol* **159**(9): 882–890.

Puska, P., J. Salonen, A. Nissinen, and J. Tuomilehto (1983). The North Karelia project. *Prev Med* **12**(1): 191–195.

Rose, G. (1981). Strategy of prevention: lessons from cardiovascular disease. *Br Med J (Clin Res Ed)* **282**(6279): 1847–1851.

Rose, G. (1985). Sick individuals and sick populations. *Int J Epidemiol* **14**(1): 32–38.

Rose, G. A., K-T. Khaw, and M. G. Marmot. (2008). *Rose's strategy of preventive medicine the complete original text*. Oxford: Oxford University Press.

4

Population Health Across Levels, Systems, and the Life Course

WE HAVE, THUS far in the book, discussed population health as a continuum and how causes of variation within a population may be distinct from causes of variation across populations. In this chapter we begin to delve into a core question in population health science: What are these "causes?"

To address this question, we begin to unpack foundational theories and models of population health, aiming not so much to provide readers with a laundry list of causes, but rather to provide frameworks that can help organize causal thinking and illuminate the hunt for causes that can be manipulated to the end of improving population health. We know intuitively that causes span multiple levels of organization, occur and accumulate across the life course in meaningful ways, and result from dynamic interactions and systems. To put it more prosaically, an individual may smoke because she likes the feeling she gets when smoking and because cigarettes are legal (individual and policy-level causes), because she started smoking when she was a teenager (a critical period for the formation of addictive behavior, illuminating causes across the life course), and because her friends smoke, giving her little motivation to quit smoking (social interactions as causes). Although no one study can capture all these sources of variation, as population health scholars we need to recognize the cascade of factors at play in determining causes of cases and causes of incidence in order to capture what matters most for population health production and to identify appropriate levers for intervention. To this end we describe three key models that inform our thinking about population health: multilevel, life course, and dynamic interactions.

1.0 Multilevel Causes of Population Health Variation

As individuals we are nested within structures with characteristics. As an obvious referent, we are all nested within families, and these families may have characteristics that influence health. For example, children who are first born have higher cognitive abilities than children born later in the birth order (Kristensen and Bjerkedal 2007), children with older siblings are at higher risk for early-onset alcohol use during adolescent years (Trim et al. 2006), and pediatric obesity risk is predicted more strongly by sibling obesity than parental obesity (Pachucki et al. 2014). Thus, family composition, number and gender of siblings, and birth order are all family-level variables that influence health, and accounting for family characteristics undoubtedly improves our ability to explain population health.

Beyond families, however, we are also nested within neighborhoods, school districts, cities, counties, states, nations, time periods, and many other levels of organization. At each of these levels, there may be exposures that occur that are ubiquitous to those within the structure but variant across structures. Consider, for example, the effect of teacher preparedness on student achievement in math. Within any classroom, we cannot measure the effect of teacher preparedness on math scores because all students have the same teacher. However, if we collect data on all classrooms in a given district, we can measure variation in teacher preparedness and correlate this with math scores. What is ubiquitous at one level (the classroom), is variant across levels (the district). This nesting within and across levels is depicted in Figure 4.1. Students are at level 1, and there may be variance in math achievement as a result of individual differences such as aptitude, amount of time spent studying, and parenting practices. These students are nested within classrooms, which is level 2. There may be variance across classrooms with respect to math achievement because of differences in teacher qualifications and teaching method, or other factors that vary across classrooms. We can also consider those classrooms nested across schools, level 3, which may indeed layer on another level of variance resulting from school resources and investments in math education. Thus, each level is nested in other levels that may contribute to variance in outcomes of interest.

Relating this to a health example, factors such as population density and urbanicity are associated with a broad range of different health indicators, including infectious disease transmission (Morse 1995, Tarwater and Martin 2001), cardiovascular disease (Yusuf et al. 2001), schizophrenia (Lewis et al. 1992, Marcelis et al. 1999, Pedersen and Mortensen 2001), and many others.

Level 1
Individual Students

Level 2
Students in Classrooms

Level 3
Classrooms in Schools

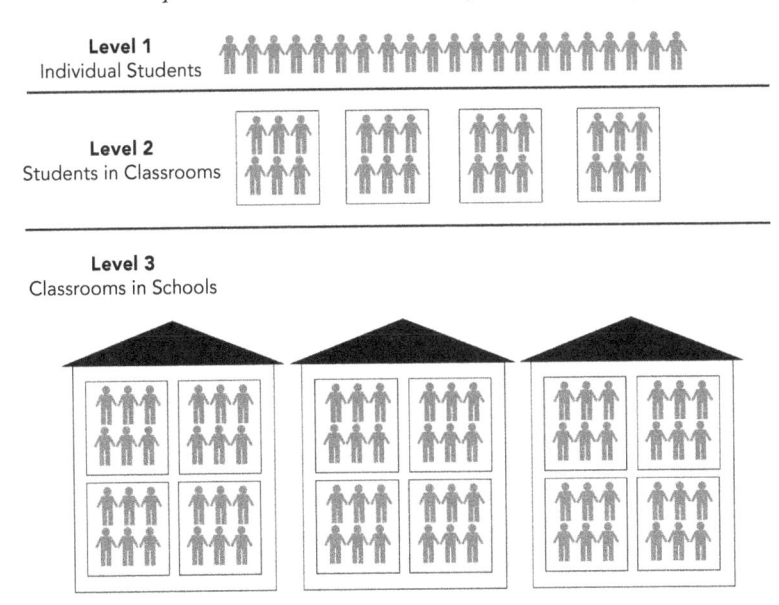

FIGURE 4.1 Example of multilevel structures in which students are nested in classrooms, which are in turn nested within schools.

Population density is ubiquitous within a particular geographic area (everyone is exposed to the same population density), but variant across areas. Thus, to understand population density and its effect on health, we need a measure of population density with enough variance that we can capture individuals in vastly different exposure levels. Other exposures with ubiquity within settings but variance across settings include factors such as road conditions, access to green space, and other civil engineering factors. States enact and enforce tobacco restrictions differently, as well as funding for prevention programs, and services for low-income families. Thus, at each level of organization in which individuals are embedded, there are numerous factors that may be important to capture and characterize to explain health both within and across each level.

A multilevel approach to population health is predicated on the understanding that exposures at many levels of organization (families, neighborhoods, cities, time periods) work together to produce health indicators. When we consider a typical or standard set of factors that may be related to health and produce variation in health status within populations—such as smoking, diet, and physical exercise—a multilevel perspective asks us to articulate the structures that produce these exposures. For example, city green space, engineering, crime, and street lighting can affect how much physical activity occurs among residents. State and local policies, convenience store density, and neighborhood social norms can indicate whether an adolescent starts smoking. Thus, we can consider these broader factors across geographic space and time as determinants of individual determinants themselves.

We can also consider the ways in which multilevel causes are structured as correlated processes through which individuals are either nested or cross-classified. An organizing framework for how to conceptualize these processes is provided in Figure 4.2. Multilevel disease occurrence includes social and economic policies that are often ubiquitous within populations but vary across populations. Furthermore, institutions and communities contain among them sets of exposures that may be influential for health. At the individual level, social relationships and individual-level risk factors such as diet, exercise, and substance use may be important determinants of individual cases and may explain across populations at least some degree of incidence variation if their prevalence differs. And, finally, the pathophysiology of disease is critical to understanding how these exposures become embedded and is essential for generating an understanding of mechanisms for disease occurrence that may be generalizable beyond specific types of exposures that may themselves be context specific.

Let us pause here to reflect on the latter point. One of the dangers of population health thinking is that we veer into the world of "miasma," or the erroneous belief in the 19th century by some prominent thinkers that disease was caused

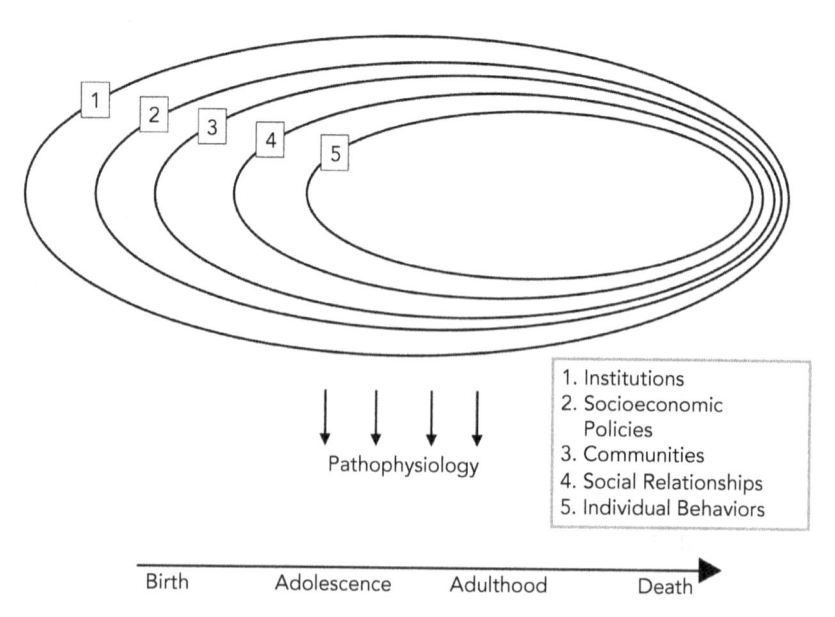

FIGURE 4.2 Causes of disease conceptualized across levels, throughout the life course, and embedded in both the social environment and pathophysiological processes.

by invisible, low-lying gases. Miasmatic thinking has us imagining that unseen forces are causing health and disease through mechanisms we do not understand. But, disease arises ultimately in individuals, and part of the purview of the population health scientist is to understand the intraindividual mechanisms through which broad structural factors produce health and disease. This is often framed as structural factors "getting under the skin" (Hatzenbuehler 2009, Hertzman and Boyce 2010, McEwen 2012), and understanding how such factors become embodied is as much of the charge to the population health scientist to investigate as are questions of whether structural factors are causally related to population health. Understanding the biology of disease occurrence—the cellular, molecular, and functional changes that occur to produce disease—and the genetic and epigenetic pathways through which exposures embed themselves is critical to the conduct of population health science.

In Box 4.1, we provide a case study in multilevel population health approaches to cardiovascular disease that evinces an understanding of how broad social structures, interpersonal relationships, individual risk factors, and variation in pathophysiology may interact to produce population rates. The case of cardiovascular disease highlights that the effects of causes in individual and social relationship levels may be embedded in causes at higher levels, and may also reflect direct relationships that occur outside those levels. For example, considering smoking as a cause of cardiovascular disease, the determinants of smoking may be embedded in higher level causes (e.g., poverty, availability), but there may be individual variation in rates and level of smoking that are not determined by higher level structures, such as genetic vulnerability to nicotine dependence and neurobiological reward pathways that reinforce the effects of smoking.

2.0 Causes of Population Health Variation Across the Life Course

Perhaps complicating matters, the multilevel causation of health in populations is not static across time, and the effects of exposures at all levels may differ depending on the life stage of the exposed. A contemplation of the dynamics of exposure occurrence across time and life stage is critical for understanding disease and health dynamics, and is considered broadly under the rubric of life course theory and practice for population health. The timing, amount, and accumulation of exposures across the life course matter, and taking into account the entire life process of exposure experiences for a population is an important part of explaining that population's health (Kuh et al. 2003).

BOX 4.1

Multilevel Approaches to Population Health Science: The Example of Cardiovascular Disease

To illustrate the potential role of multilevel thinking on our understanding of health in populations, we draw on the example of coronary heart disease (CHD), the leading cause of death in the United States (610,000 per year), responsible for approximately one quarter of all annual deaths (Centers for Disease Control and Prevention 2015b). CHD has been studied largely in relation to diet (Mente et al. 2009), physical activity (Li and Siegrist 2012), and smoking (Huxley and Woodward 2011), each of which are critical and modifiable factors that are indeed associated with CHD. Yet, if we focus only on these exposures, we risk confinement to the proximate prison of risk-factor epidemiology (McMichael 1999), missing the levels of public health impact that lie at "higher" levels of organization. During the past two decades, the study of CHD has extended to neighborhood-level social environments (Chaix 2009). For example, the socioeconomic environment is associated with CHD incidence, with greater neighborhood disadvantage predicting higher incidence (Diez Roux et al. 2001), beyond individual risk factors, among both blacks and whites. In particular, neighborhood median housing value is related inversely to hypertension (a risk factor for CHD) among black women, independent of individual-level risk factors. Similarly, neighborhood-level social capital is a predictor of CHD mortality (Chaix 2009). Therefore, the drivers of CHD rest both at the individual and group levels, being well in line with a multilevel perspective on the production of population health.

Extending this example, from 1979 through 2009, CHD mortality declined by 66% among men and 67% among women (Ford et al. 2014) (see Figure 4.3). However, these general gains mask differences by race, which emerge clearly in Figure 4.4, showing that despite the overall reduction in CHD mortality, the rates for black men and women remain disproportionately highest relative to other race/gender groupings (Ford et al. 2014).

Why would this be?

Informed by a multilevel perspective, one could approach this question in a few ways. Can genomic differences explain racial disparities in CHD? Ample evidence suggests that genomic factors do not appear to explain racial disparities in population-level CHD burden (Kaufman et al. 2015). Could this difference be related to disparities in access to and quality of care

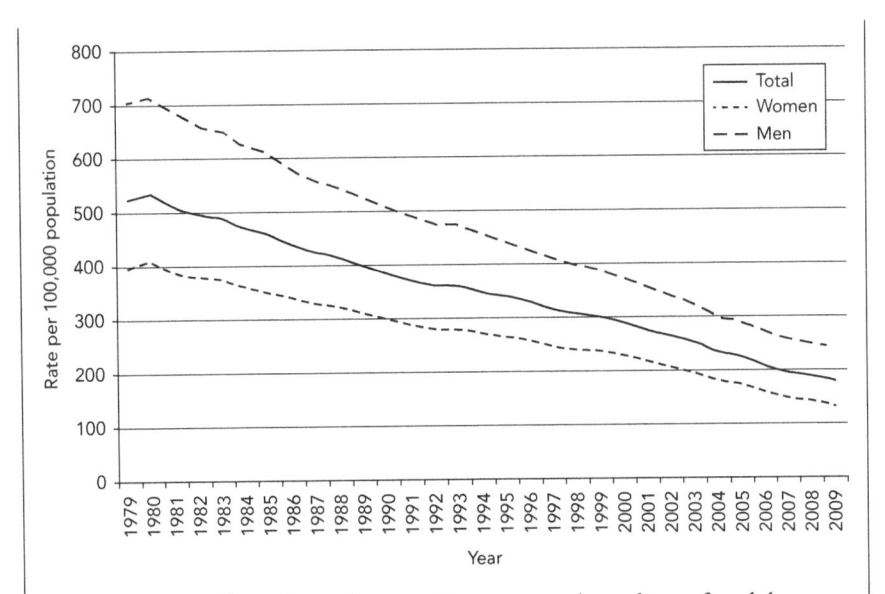

FIGURE 4.3 Age-adjusted mortality rates from coronary heart disease for adults 25 years or older in the United States.

Source: Ford, E. S., V. L. Roger, S. M. Dunlay, A. S. Go, and W. D. Rosamond. (2014). "Challenges of ascertaining national trends in the incidence of coronary heart disease in the United States." *J Am Heart Assoc* **3**(6): e001097.

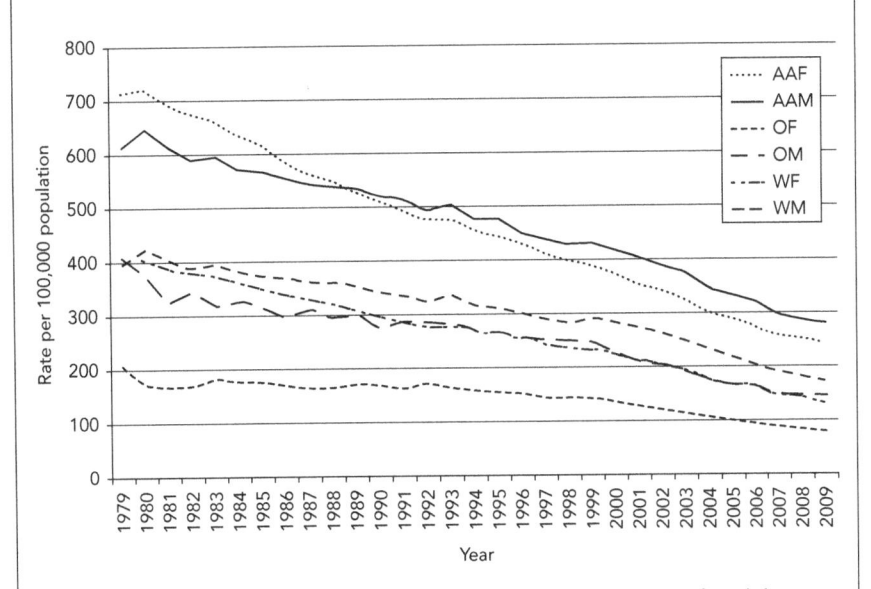

FIGURE 4.4 Age-adjusted mortality rates from coronary heart disease for adults 25 years or older by race and gender in the United States. AAF, African American females; AAM, African American males; OF, other females; OM, other males; WF, white females; WM, white males.

Source: Ford, E. S., V. L. Roger, S. M. Dunlay, A. S. Go, and W. D. Rosamond. (2014). "Challenges of ascertaining national trends in the incidence of coronary heart disease in the United States." *J Am Heart Assoc* **3**(6): e001097.

(Graham 2014)? Perhaps, although the best available evidence suggests disparities in access to and quality of care are likely to explain relatively little of these observed racial differences.

Extending a multilevel lens, an exploration of the geographic differences in disparities in CHD by race shows that although mortality is higher for blacks than whites at any level of urbanization, there are substantial regional differences by race (Kulshreshtha et al. 2014). For example, among blacks in the United States in 2009, the highest rate of CHD mortality was found in midwestern rural areas (231 per 100,000), whereas the lowest rate was found in northeastern rural areas (147 per 100,000). In contrast, among whites, the highest rate of CHD mortality was found among large metro areas in the Northeast (192 per 100,000) whereas the lowest rate was found in medium-size metro areas in the West (134 per 100,000). Could "higher level" group determinants of CHD, then, better explain racial differences in CHD? A geographically weighted regression approach demonstrated that geographic heterogeneity in black–white differences in CHD mortality was attributable both to poverty and segregation (Gebreab and Diez Roux 2012). After controlling for poverty, segregation was associated positively with CHD for blacks in some counties and associated negatively with CHD in others, suggesting its significance differs by place. Variation in features of the built environment, including "walkability" and air pollution (Hankey et al. 2012), is also associated jointly with CHD mortality. Thus, in addition to approaching racial disparities in CHD by promoting equal access to quality health care, we would also do well to consider economic deprivation and segregation as key targets of study and intervention.

This illustration demonstrates how an exploration of influences at multiple levels can shed light much more comprehensively on the determinants of population health than a focus on single levels alone.

We acknowledge the work of Gregory Cohen, MSW, on the material in this box.

Centrally, life course approaches attempt to assess how exposures arise and produce health throughout life, and how we make sense of these interconnected temporal processes. The scope of specific factors that vary across the life course in time and importance includes, for example, physical growth, social mobility, behavior changes, physical environment, and life role transitions. Life course approaches also extend beyond the life of any one individual to suggest connections in health across generations. Considering a life course approach to mental health would guide use toward questions not only about the conditions in adulthood that increase risk for poor mental health, but also experiences such as childhood exposures to traumatic events change later risk for mental health problems. It would also have us consider how parental and grandparental social and life circumstances set a course for the development of poor mental health in future generations. A life course perspective suggests that we cannot ignore these important questions. Unless we understand the traumatic events experienced during childhood, and the circumstances of parents and grandparents, our understanding of poor mental health in adulthood is going to remain limited and incomplete.

The recognition that life staging matters for exposure occurrence may seem an obvious need for population health science, especially for those who have studied developmental psychology or biology. However, the development of life course population health as a subdiscipline of health science traces its roots to medicine and epidemiology, which was predominately concerned throughout the mid to late 20th century with exposures that occur in adulthood—particularly diet, exercise, and smoking—and their impacts on chronic disease such as cardiovascular disease and cancer. The development of life course theory is often attributed to research developed and advanced by David Barker, who championed the theory that causes of cardiovascular disease can be traced back to in utero and infant exposure (Barker 1995, Barker 1997, Barker 1999). His work documented that factors such as birth weight and other neonatal factors are associated with the development of cardiovascular disease in adulthood, suggesting there is fetal and early life programming that occurs but may not manifest for decades of life. Although a debate remains regarding the importance of such neonatal growth factors for cardiovascular disease, Barker's research was a catalyst that led to the recognition that there may be many such early-life origins of adult disease (Lawlor et al. 2003, Lynch and Smith 2005, Smith 2007, Naess et al. 2008), including exposures that occur and embed but do not exert an effect for years or even decades, as well as research that as explicated the various mechanisms through which early-life exposures may influence current and later health of populations.

Within the life course framework, we present here three basic processes through which exposures may influence disease risk (Figure 4.5). We discuss these processes to provide a general background and tool kit to approach the understanding of population health by considering whether the production of health may be the result of one or more of these processes: critical/sensitive periods for exposure occurrence, chains of risk, and accumulation of exposure. These processes are not mutually exclusive, and

Critical/Sensitive Period
In a critical or sensitive period model, exposures occurring during a specific developmental stage influence health indicators. The influence of the exposure on the health indicator can be latent; an exposure occurring in utero or in infancy can manifest effects in adulthood, for example.

Critical Period

(In Utero) Birth Early Childhood Adolescence Adulthood Older Age → Disease Onset

Chains of Risk
In a chains of risk model, exposures occurring early during the life course influence the occurrence and magnitude of other exposures throughout development. Thus, risk A has an influence on health by changing the probability of exposure to risk B, which in turn influences the probability of exposure to risk C, and so forth.

Risk A → Risk B → Risk C → Risk D

(In Utero) Birth Early Childhood Adolescence Adulthood Older Age → Disease Onset

Accumulation of Risk
In the accumulation of risk model, health indicators are caused by the combination of risks that accumulate throughout the life course. For example, an exposure that occurs in infancy may not be sufficient to influence a health indicator, but the combination of an exposure in infancy, another exposure in childhood, and another exposure in early adulthood, may work together to influence health indicators. These exposures could be acute (e.g., traumatic brain injury at a young age) or chronic (e.g., pack-years of smoking).

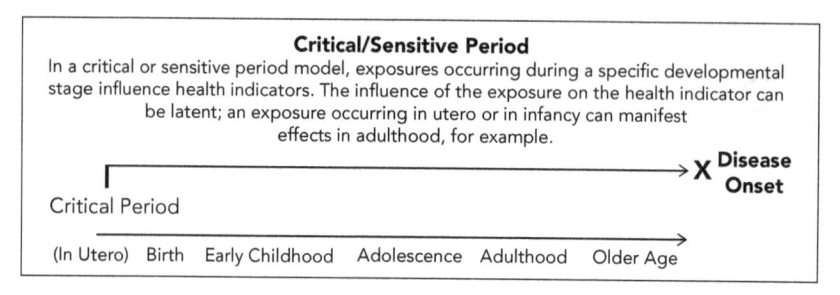

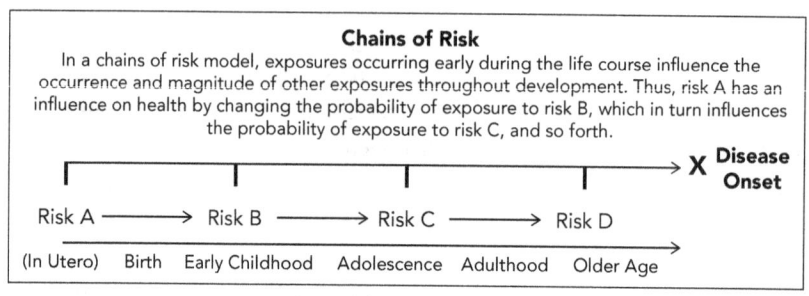

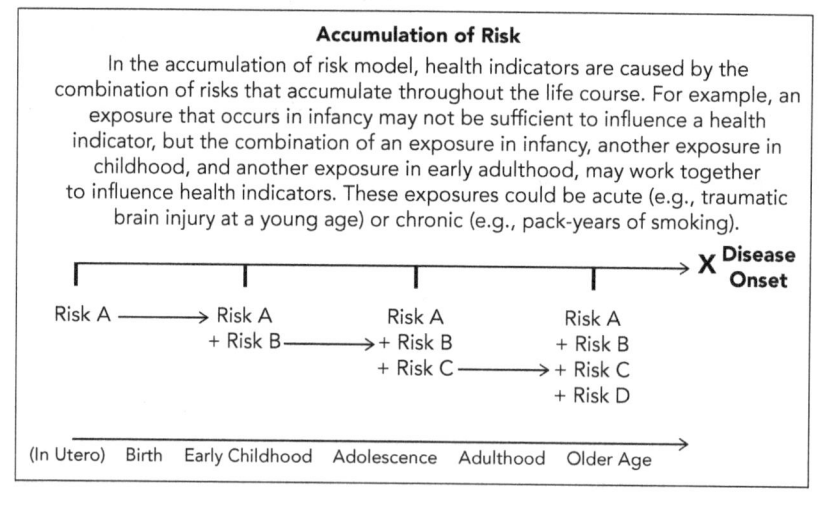

Risk A → Risk A + Risk B → Risk A + Risk B + Risk C → Risk A + Risk B + Risk C + Risk D

(In Utero) Birth Early Childhood Adolescence Adulthood Older Age → Disease Onset

FIGURE 4.5 Three core models that may explain life course influences on population health.

for any particular health outcome there may be several of these processes occurring, or none. Furthermore, these pathways are not the only ones through which exposures that occur across the life course may influence disease development. These models as well as others have been explicated in much greater detail in texts devoted to life course processes. We refer readers to other work (Kuh et al. 2003, 2014) for a more in-depth discussion of life course approaches.

2.1 Critical/Sensitive Periods

The same exposure experienced during utero, infancy, childhood, or adulthood may have different effects on health. However, there are cases when an exposure exerts an effect on a particular health indicator principally during a single developmental period. In these cases, this period is said to be a *critical period*. An exposure that has a greater effect during one stage of the life course than another stage is often said to be a *sensitive period*. Thus, while linked, a critical period is one in which exposure occurrence will *only* have an effect if occurring during the developmental period, whereas a sensitive period is one in which exposure occurrence will have a *greater* effect if occurring during the developmental period, but will have present albeit lesser effects if occurring in other developmental stages.

The in utero environment is an intuitive example of the critical/sensitive period. Rapid changes and growth are occurring in a developing fetus, especially in comparison with any other stage of life outside the womb. Furthermore, the fetus is entirely dependent on nutrients and oxygen from the mother, and even low exposure to toxins that would be safe for children and adults can render increased risks of complications to the developing fetus.

There are several prominent examples of the in utero environment as a critical period for the developing fetus. For example, a common treatment believed to reduce risk for miscarriage was a prescription for diethylstilbestrol (DES), a synthetic estrogen hormone. DES was given to many pregnant women during the 1950s and 1960s. Daughters of these women demonstrated demonstrably higher incidence of vaginal cancer, which usually manifested during their teenage years (Herbst et al. 1971). Other adverse health indicators for both daughters and sons of DES-exposed women have been documented, and potential effects on the third generation are now being investigated. Thus, exposure to DES in utero, during a period of rapid development, was influential in the development of vaginal cancer, but decades after the exposure occurred. As another example, Susser and Lin (1992) examined the offspring of women exposed to famine during the Nazi blockade of western Holland during the World War II. Adults who were in the first trimester of gestation at the time of the most severe part of the famine were at increased risk for neurodevelopmental disorders, including schizophrenia. Thus, first trimester of gestation was a critical period for the development of health indicators in adulthood due to deprivation of nutrition during that window (Susser and Lin 1992, Brown et al. 1995, Susser et al. 1996).

Critical and sensitive periods are not only confined to the in utero experience, however. The terms have been used in developmental psychology and learning for decades to describe the importance of early life as the center stage for brain development and the potential long-lasting effects of deprivation during this time for many later outcomes. Such critical/sensitive periods may occur throughout the life course for specific exposures and specific outcomes; thus, considering the important developmental windows for exposure occurrence is critical for population health.

One of the most important aspects of critical/sensitive periods is the potential long latency between the occurrence of the exposure and its effects. This fact can hamper study designs to investigate the effects of early-life exposures on later health, because the long latency times require long follow-up periods to observe health indicators. Furthermore, the multitude of exposures that occur after the focal exposure and the methods to estimate their effects create conceptual and analytic challenges. However, birth cohort studies that monitor and measure pregnancy and early-life exposure and their relationship to adult health are growing in number, and methods to estimate such effects are developing at rapid pace, incorporating traditional cohort methods along with methods to estimate time-varying confounding, mediation, and more complex modeling strategies.

2.2   Chains of Risk

Although the experience of certain exposures during a specific developmental period may affect the risk for various health indicators directly, a life course approach also acknowledges that exposures themselves are often embedded in a causal sequence that may lead to the development of an adverse health outcome.

For example, although high blood pressure in adulthood is a risk factor for the development of cardiovascular disease, a chains of risk model may explicate the preceding causes of the high blood pressure itself. For example, being born into deprived social circumstances may result in inadequate nutrition at an early age, which may lead to childhood obesity, which may reinforce poor eating behaviors and a sedentary lifestyle, which may affect future earning and job placement, residential mobility, social status in adulthood, and ultimately the development of high blood pressure, which places individuals at risk for cardiovascular disease. Such a model has been proposed by Kuh and Ben-Shlomo (2004) and others as an explanation for the ways in which prenatal and early-life socioeconomic position and deprivation may influence adult chronic disease. Thus, we might consider early-life deprivation to be a cause of adulthood cardiovascular disease mediated by a chain of factors that included health behaviors and intermediate health conditions, all of which together were causally related and led to the development of cardiovascular disease.

One powerful way in which the chains of risk model can be interpreted is by considering the most efficient ways in which we can affect adult health. The model suggests that the risk factors proximal to the onset of disease events in adulthood, such as diet, substance use, and obesity, are the products of a lifetime of accumulation of exposures. Intervening earlier during the life course may prevent a cascade of health problems that are difficult to retract in adulthood, when habits have been formed and community roots have been laid. By focusing on health promotion at the earliest ages, we may be able to realize a profound impact on population health in adulthood. Practically, however, such efforts have been met with hesitation. The results of early-intervention work cannot be observed for decades, and as such requires substantial investment with no immediate results in many cases. Nonetheless, a chains of risk model is an important reminder to investigate the ways in which exposures in adulthood arise, and it forces us to think about intervention points during the life course when the greatest good can occur.

2.3 Accumulation of Risk

In contrast to the chains of risk model, in which one exposure causes another exposure and in totality mediate the emergence of health problems, the accumulation of risk model is one in which exposures may not be related causally to each other, but together affect disease risk as they accumulate throughout the life course. For example, for some people, a single traumatic experience during childhood may not cause the development of mental or physical health problems in adulthood; however, a lifetime of accumulating traumatic experiences from childhood to adulthood may be enough of a "tipping point" to cause a mental or physical health incident. Accumulation of risk across the life course can refer both to exposures that are similar in categorization (e.g., continuing to smoke from adolescence through adulthood, chronic exposure to discrimination resulting from marginalized social status) or the accumulation of exposures that are distinct but together work to produce the outcome (e.g., early-life deprivation, experience of trauma, unemployment and financial strain, childhood and adolescent health problems). The central thesis of the accumulation of risk model is that as we progress through the life course, we collect the summation of life experience and exposures we encounter. These exposures can amass to a point after which adverse health indicators may occur. Thus, the accumulation of risk model can be viewed as the interaction among exposures as they occur throughout the life course, in contrast to the chains of risk model in which one exposure leads to another exposure.

Drawing from the psychiatric epidemiological literature as an example, there is growing evidence that stressful exposures throughout the life course generate such an accumulation of risk approach. Although it is well known that exposure to a traumatic experience during adulthood increases the risk of subsequent psychopathology (Kessler et al. 1995), there is substantial individual variation in who becomes ill after such traumatic exposures. Accumulating evidence indicates that exposure to stressors during childhood, such as abuse and neglect, death of a parent, or other potentially traumatic experiences, potentiate the effects of stress experiences during adulthood (McLaughlin et al. 2010a). That is, those who are at highest risk for development of psychopathology after a traumatic event are those who experienced trauma as children. These potentiated pathways may be mediated by several psychological mechanisms, including dysregulation in physiological stress response systems (Heim and Nemeroff 2001), increase in emotional reactivity (Wichers et al. 2009, McLaughlin et al. 2010b), and disruptions in the ability to modulate negative emotions adaptively (McLaughlin and Hatzenbuehler 2009). This is an accumulation of risk model; as adverse experiences accumulate throughout the life course, individuals become increasingly more likely to develop psychopathology with each additional stressor.

2.4 Summary of the Life Course Models

In Table 4.1 we provide a summary of the three models. We can conceptualize critical/sensitive period effects as direct effects of exposure on outcome, we can conceptualize chains of risk as effects of exposure on outcome mediated by other exposures, and we can conceptualize accumulation of risk as effects of exposure interacting with or moderating other exposures. As such, life course approaches to population health are similar to many other analyses we conduct in population health science: we select exposures and outcomes of interest and then examine direct effects, mediators, and moderators of that relationship. The difference embedded in life course approaches to population health is in the explicit theory and incorporation of early-life exposures as well as those that occur during critical developmental life stages.

We emphasize that these three approaches are not the only approaches to studying health across the life course, but argue they are the fundamental approaches. With these conceptual frameworks in mind, population health scientists can engage in a critical examination of both the structural processes that generate observed data patterns across populations as well as the cross-generational and life course exposures through which population patterns emerge and are transmitted at all levels of organization.

Table 4.1 Life Course Approaches to Population Health Science

Life Course Approach	Definition of Analytic Feature	Example
Critical/sensitive periods	There is a direct effect of exposure on the outcome.	Examples include DES exposure in utero and vaginal cancer in adolescence (Herbst et al. 1971), nutritional deprivation in utero and neurodevelopmental disorders in adulthood (Susser and Lin 1992), and substance use during early adolescence and a later risk for psychiatric disorders (Grant and Dawson 1997).
Chains of risk	Exposure affects the outcome by causing other exposures.	Early life deprivation and later chronic disease may be mediated during adulthood by influencing health behaviors, education, and geographic location (Kuh and Ben-Shlomo 2004).
Accumulation of risk	Exposure affects outcome through interaction with other exposures that accumulate during the life course.	Early-life traumatic events influence the development of psychiatric disorders to a greater extent among those who are then exposed to later traumatic events (McLaughlin et al. 2010a, 2010b; Sheridan and McLaughlin 2014).

DES, diethylstilbestrol.

3.0 Dynamic Interactions and Population Health Variation

A third theoretical framework that must be considered for population health science to flourish centers around the dynamic systems through which exposures are embedded and health occurs. To understand the utility of systems approaches to population health, consider a typical approach to assessment of distribution and determinants. Within a population, we collect data on a set of risk factors and use group comparison as well as regression-based approaches to estimate the correlation between the exposure and the outcome, first unadjusted and then perhaps adjusted for a set of hypothesized confounders. Assumptions embedded for the validity of these models include, among others, that there is no interference between units (i.e., the disease status of person A does not affect the exposure status of person B), that individuals are independent (e.g., all residual error after model estimation is random, with an expectation of zero), and that there are no discontinuous nonlinear relations that are unaccounted for in the model (Kleinbaum 2008).

Such assumptions are unlikely to hold when examining the processes through which population health arises. As a clear example, consider the emergence of influenza in a population. Influenza is an infectious disease spread from person to person through physical contact with an infected person. Therefore, understanding the causes of influenza requires not only comparison of those affected and those unaffected, but also theoretical frameworks that acknowledge and model the interdependencies and networks through which affected and susceptible individuals come into contact. The cases of influenza within a particular community are not independent; they *cannot* be independent because each individual must come into contact with an infected person. In fact, systems approaches to the investigation of transmission patterns of disease for communicable infections have been part of population health science for many decades, in various forms. The use of complex computational models to understand social network mixing patterns for HIV transmission and other sexually transmitted diseases has illuminated the ways in which mixing patterns can generate epidemics, the dynamics of transmission based on characteristics of networks, and the best and most efficacious control strategies to reduce the reproductive rate of disease.

More broadly, population health science increasingly acknowledges that understanding the production of health requires an approach that recognizes the ways in which individuals are embedded in systems within which individuals interact with each other and their environments. Population health is the product of a complex system of interrelated factors that produce health through dynamic processes, characterized by interrelations, nonlinearity, reciprocity, and emergence. Therefore, although system simplification can yield important insights that can inform public health efforts, increasingly we are recognizing unintended consequences of oversimplification of complex systems, suggesting that a complex systems conceptual lens, perhaps supplemented by complex systems analytic approaches, can be a useful part of our public health armamentarium. A traditional approach of identifying associations between risk factors and health indicators, even if these associations are across levels and the life course, may not take into account the full range of factors that may influence population distributions of health. Thus, we are required in many circumstances to adopt a complex systems lens and relevant methods of analysis.

There are several prominent examples of such systems approaches in the epidemiological literature that serve as exemplars for the types of systems approaches we advocate in this chapter. Obesity, for example, remains a health outcome that is of central interest in population health science because the prevalence continues to be high in many countries, and efforts to reduce obesity have stalled. Systems approaches to understanding the spread and dynamics of obesity have fueled important population health insights. For example, Christakis and Fowler (2007) demonstrated an association between weight gain within social networks and the impact on individual risk for subsequent weight gain using a population-based sample with decades of follow-up information. Although the methods and inference have attracted some controversy (e.g., see Cohen-Cole and Fletcher 2008), the empirical incorporation of social network modeling and systems approaches to understanding population health patterns is an important methodological and substantive development for the field. Other approaches to systems science with regard to obesity have used computational modeling to demonstrate the importance of school and social networks, food outlets and choices, food policy, and food supply (Levy et al. 2011), and other macro- and individual-level factors that are dynamic over time and exert influence by becoming embedded within communities that are themselves reflections of broader social networks.

In summary, although the process of weight gain involves calorie intake and accretion, the underlying causal architecture behind how BMI and obesity are distributed across populations requires an understanding of multilevel, life course, and systems processes. Food supply, food outlets, network mixing patterns, family composition, schools, peer groups, and many other factors that are not independent within and across populations influence how obesity arises. A systems approach is being used increasingly in population health science with regard to obesity to demonstrate the drivers of these outcomes at the population level. Such systems approaches are used to characterize violence and other injury outcomes (Cerda et al. 2015), HIV transmission and treatment patterns (Westreich et al. 2012), obesity and other cardiometabolic outcomes (El-Sayed et al. 2013), and many other health indicators of importance for population health worldwide.

Importantly, failing to conceptualize population health systems as complex systems can lead to unintended consequences. For example, efforts at cutting cigarette nicotine levels (National Cancer Institute 2001) can lead to compensatory smoking, illustrating the unanticipated consequences of particular system perturbations if we do not consider the system's dimensions and interrelations completely. Similar examples of consequences of simple systems approaches include antiretroviral therapy prolonging the lives of HIV carriers but potentially leading to HIV spread as a result of lower risk perception (Cassell et al. 2006), antibiotic overuse worsening pathogen resistance (Centers for Disease Control and Prevention 2015a), antilock brakes leading to more risky driving (Winston et al. 2006), and use of protective headgear in football failing to decrease concussions as a result of risk compensation (Daneshvar, Baugh et al. 2011).

Therefore, at its core, complex systems thinking brings to population health science an appreciation of the interconnectedness of elements of population systems that both determine and are determined by health indicators. Analytically, there are several methods that can be applied to the analysis of complex systems, including agent-based modeling, (Marshall and Galea 2015), network modeling (Luke and Harris 2007), and the parametric g-formula (Hernan 2015). These methods have allowed us to conceptualize and analyze population health as a dynamic system, to analyze more realistically the drivers of health, and to explore the potential effects of population approaches to disease prevention.

4.0 Summary

The production of health in populations arises from causes at multiple levels of organization—from the societal level and through social policy to communities and families—and manifests through interindividual variation in genetic and molecular factors that influence susceptibility and progression. This process leads to our fourth principle of population health science (Box 4.2).

Causes that matter for health occur throughout the life course, and health distributions within population arise as a result of dynamic interactions of individuals with their environments. Theoretical models, analytic techniques, and empirical demonstrations of feasibility have generated tremendous

---

BOX 4.2

Fourth foundational principle of population health science

The causes of population health are multilevel, accumulate throughout the life course, and are embedded in dynamic interpersonal relationships.

growth and promise in the incorporation of multilevel, life course, and dynamic systems approaches to data analysis and interpretation. These theories and their analytic offshoots are fundamental interconnected parts of a robust population health science, pushing population health scientists to consider the routes through we may best understand the production of population health so we may intervene to improve it.

5.0 References

Barker, D. J. (1995). Fetal origins of coronary heart disease. *BMJ* **311**(6998): 171–174.

Barker, D. J. (1997). Maternal nutrition, fetal nutrition, and disease in later life. *Nutrition* **13**(9): 807–813.

Barker, D. J. (1999). Early growth and cardiovascular disease. *Arch Dis Child* **80**(4): 305–307.

Brown, A. S., E. S. Susser, S. P. Lin, R. Neugebauer, and J. M. Gorman. (1995). Increased risk of affective disorders in males after second trimester prenatal exposure to the Dutch hunger winter of 1944–45. *Br J Psychiatry* **166**(5): 601–606.

Cassell, M. M., D. T. Halperin, J. D. Shelton, and D. Stanton. (2006). Risk compensation: the Achilles' heel of innovations in HIV prevention? *BMJ* **332**(7541): 605–607.

Centers for Disease Control and Prevention. (2015a). *Centers for Disease Control and Prevention, Antibiotic/Antimicrobial Resistance*. Available at: www.cdc.gov/drugresistance/. Accessed April 22, 2016.

Centers for Disease Control and Prevention. (2015b). *Heart disease statistics and maps*. Available: http://www.cdc.gov/heartdisease/facts.htm.

Cerda, M., M. Tracy, K. M. Keyes, and S. Galea. (2015). To treat or to prevent?: reducing the population burden of violence-related post-traumatic stress disorder. *Epidemiology* **26**(5): 681–689.

Chaix, B. (2009). Geographic life environments and coronary heart disease: a literature review, theoretical contributions, methodological updates, and a research agenda. *Annu Rev Public Health* **30**: 81–105.

Christakis, N., and J. Fowler. (2007). The spread of obesity in a large social network over 32 years. *N Engl J Med* **357**: 370–379.

Cohen-Cole, E., and J. M. Fletcher. (2008). Is obesity contagious? Social networks vs. environmental factors in the obesity epidemic. *J Health Econ* **27**(5): 1382–1387.

Daneshvar, D. H., C. M. Baugh, C. J. Nowinski, A. C. McKee, R. A. Stern, and R. C. Cantu. (2011). Helmets and mouth guards: the role of personal equipment in preventing sport-related concussions. *Clin Sports Med* **30**(1): 145–163, x.

Diez Roux, A. V., S. S. Merkin, D. Arnett, L. Chambless, M. Massing, F. J. Nieto, et al. (2001). Neighborhood of residence and incidence of coronary heart disease. *N Engl J Med* **345**(2): 99–106.

El-Sayed, A. M., L. Seemann, P. Scarborough, and S. Galea. (2013). Are network-based interventions a useful antiobesity strategy? An application of simulation models for causal inference in epidemiology. *Am J Epidemiol* **178**(2): 287–295.

Ford, E. S., V. L. Roger, S. M. Dunlay, A. S. Go, and W. D. Rosamond. (2014). Challenges of ascertaining national trends in the incidence of coronary heart disease in the United States. *J Am Heart Assoc* **3**(6): e001097.

Gebreab, S. Y., and A. V. Diez Roux. (2012). Exploring racial disparities in CHD mortality between blacks and whites across the United States: a geographically weighted regression approach. *Health Place* **18**(5): 1006–1014.

Graham, G. (2014). Population-based approaches to understanding disparities in cardiovascular disease risk in the United States. *Int J Gen Med* **7**: 393–400.

Grant, B. F., and D. A. Dawson (1997). Age at onset of alcohol use and its association with DSM-IV alcohol abuse and dependence: results from the National Longitudinal Alcohol Epidemiologic Survey. *J Subst Abuse* **9**: 103–110.

Hankey, S., J. D. Marshall, and M. Brauer. (2012). Health impacts of the built environment: within-urban variability in physical inactivity, air pollution, and ischemic heart disease mortality. *Environ Health Perspect* **120**(2): 247–253.

Hatzenbuehler, M. L. (2009). How does sexual minority stigma 'get under the skin?' A psychological mediation framework. *Psychol Bull* **135**(5): 707–730.

Heim, C., and C. B. Nemeroff. (2001). The role of childhood trauma in the neurobiology of mood and anxiety disorders: preclinical and clinical studies. *Biol Psychiatry* **49**(12): 1023–1039.

Herbst, A. L., H. Ulfelder, and D. C. Poskanzer. (1971). Adenocarcinoma of the vagina: association of maternal stilbestrol therapy with tumor appearance in young women. *N Engl J Med* **284**(15): 878–881.

Hernan, M. A. (2015). Invited commentary: Agent-based models for causal inference: reweighting data and theory in epidemiology. *Am J Epidemiol* **181**(2): 103–105.

Hertzman, C., and T. Boyce. (2010). How experience gets under the skin to create gradients in developmental health. *Annu Rev Public Health* **31**: 329–347.

Huxley, R. R., and M. Woodward. (2011). Cigarette smoking as a risk factor for coronary heart disease in women compared with men: a systematic review and meta-analysis of prospective cohort studies. *Lancet* **378**(9799): 1297–1305.

Kaufman, J. S., L. Dolman, D. Rushani, and R. S. Cooper. (2015). The contribution of genomic research to explaining racial disparities in cardiovascular disease: a systematic review. *Am J Epidemiol* **181**(7): 464–472.

Kessler, R. C., A. Sonnega, E. Bromet, M. Hughes, and C. B. Nelson. (1995). Posttraumatic stress disorder in the National Comorbidity Survey. *Arch Gen Psychiatry* **52**(12): 1048–1060.

Kleinbaum, D. G. (2008). *Applied regression analysis and other multivariable methods.* Belmont, CA: Thomson Brooks/Cole Publishing.

Kristensen, P., and T. Bjerkedal. (2007). Explaining the relation between birth order and intelligence. *Science* **316**(5832): 1717.

Kuh, D., and Y. Ben-Shlomo. (2004). Socioeconomic pathways between childhood and adult health. In *A life course approach to chronic disease epidemiology*. D. Kuh, Y. Ben-Shlomo, and E. Susser, editors. Oxford: Oxford University Press: 371–395.

Kuh, D., Y. Ben-Shlomo, J. Lynch, J. Hallqvist, and C. Power. (2003). Life course epidemiology. *J Epidemiol Community Health* **57**(10): 778–783.

Kuh, D., R. Cooper, R. Hardy, M. Richards, and Y. Ben-Shlomo. (2014). *A life course approach to healthy ageing.* Oxford, UK: Oxford University Press.

Kulshreshtha, A., A. Goyal, K. Dabhadkar, E. Veledar, and V. Vaccarino. (2014). Urban–rural differences in coronary heart disease mortality in the United States: 1999–2009. *Public Health Rep* **129**(1): 19–29.

Lawlor, D. A., S. Ebrahim, and G. D. Smith. (2003). The association of socio-economic position across the life course and age at menopause: the British Women's Heart and Health Study. *BJOG* **110**(12): 1078–1087.

Levy, D. T., P. L. Mabry, Y. C. Wang, S. Gortmaker, T. T. Huang, T. Marsh, et al. (2011). Simulation models of obesity: a review of the literature and implications for research and policy. *Obes Rev* **12**(5): 378–394.

Lewis, G., A. David, S. Andreasson, and P. Allebeck. (1992). Schizophrenia and city life. *Lancet* **340**(8812): 137–140.

Li, J., and J. Siegrist. (2012). Physical activity and risk of cardiovascular disease: a meta-analysis of prospective cohort studies. *Int J Environ Res Public Health* **9**(2): 391–407.

Luke, D. A., and J. K. Harris. (2007). Network analysis in public health: history, methods, and applications. *Annu Rev Public Health* **28**: 69–93.

Lynch, J., and G. D. Smith. (2005). A life course approach to chronic disease epidemiology. *Annu Rev Public Health* **26**: 1–35.

Marcelis, M., N. Takei, and J. van Os. (1999). Urbanization and risk for schizophrenia: does the effect operate before or around the time of illness onset? *Psychol Med* **29**(5): 1197–1203.

Marshall, B. D., and S. Galea. (2015). Formalizing the role of agent-based modeling in causal inference and epidemiology. *Am J Epidemiol* **181**(2): 92–99.

McEwen, B. S. (2012). Brain on stress: how the social environment gets under the skin. *Proc Natl Acad Sci U S A* **109**(Suppl 2): 17180–17185.

McLaughlin, K. A., K. J. Conron, K. C. Koenen, and S. E. Gilman. (2010a). Childhood adversity, adult stressful life events, and risk of past-year psychiatric disorder: a test of the stress sensitization hypothesis in a population-based sample of adults. *Psychol Med* **40**(10): 1647–1658.

McLaughlin, K. A., and M. L. Hatzenbuehler. (2009). Mechanisms linking stressful life events and mental health problems in a prospective, community-based sample of adolescents. *J Adolesc Health* **44**(2): 153–160.

McLaughlin, K. A., L. D. Kubzansky, E. C. Dunn, R. Waldinger, G. Vaillant, and K. C. Koenen. (2010b). Childhood social environment, emotional reactivity to stress, and mood and anxiety disorders across the life course. *Depress Anxiety* **27**(12): 1087–1094.

McMichael, A. J. (1999). Prisoners of the proximate: loosening the constraints on epidemiology in an age of change. *Am J Epidemiol* **149**(10): 887–897.

Mente, A., L. de Koning, H. S. Shannon, and S. S. Anand. (2009). A systematic review of the evidence supporting a causal link between dietary factors and coronary heart disease. *Arch Intern Med* **169**(7): 659–669.

Morse, S. S. (1995). Factors in the emergence of infectious diseases. *Emerg Infect Dis* **1**(1): 7–15.

Naess, O., B. Claussen, G. D. Smith, and A. H. Leyland. (2008). Life course influence of residential area on cause-specific mortality. *J Epidemiol Community Health* **62**(1): 29–34.

National Cancer Institute. (2001). *Risks associated with smoking cigarettes with low machine-measured yields of tar and nicotine.* Bethesda, MD: U.S. Department of Health and Human Services, Public Health Service, National Institutes of Health, National Cancer Institute.

Pachucki, M. C., M. F. Lovenheim, and M. Harding. (2014). Within-family obesity associations: evaluation of parent, child, and sibling relationships. *Am J Prev Med* **47**(4): 382–391.

Pedersen, C., and P. Mortensen. (2001). Evidence of a dose–response relationship between urbanicity during upbringing and schizophrenia risk. *Arch Gen Psychiatry* **58**(11): 1039–1046.

Sheridan, M. A., and K. A. McLaughlin. (2014). Dimensions of early experience and neural development: deprivation and threat. *Trends Cogn Sci* **18**(11): 580–585.

Smith, G. D. (2007). Life-course approaches to inequalities in adult chronic disease risk. *Proc Nutr Soc* **66**(2): 216–236.

Susser, E. S., and S. P. Lin. (1992). Schizophrenia after prenatal exposure to the Dutch Hunger Winter of 1944–1945. *Arch Gen Psychiatry* **49**(12): 983–988.

Susser, E., R. Neugebauer, H. W. Hoek, A. S. Brown, S. Lin, D. Labovitz, et al. (1996). Schizophrenia after prenatal famine: further evidence. *Arch Gen Psychiatry* **53**(1): 25–31.

Tarwater, P. M., and C. F. Martin. (2001). Effects of population density on the spread of disease. *Complexity* **6**(6): 29–36.

Trim, R. S., E. Leuthe, and L. Chassin. (2006). Sibling influence on alcohol use in a young adult, high-risk sample. *J Stud Alcohol* **67**(3): 391–398.

Westreich, D., S. R. Cole, J. G. Young, F. Palella, P. C. Tien, L. Kingsley, et al. (2012). The parametric g-formula to estimate the effect of highly active antiretroviral therapy on incident AIDS or death. *Stat Med* **31**(18): 2000–2009.

Wichers, M., N. Geschwind, N. Jacobs, G. Kenis, F. Peeters, C. Derom, et al. (2009). Transition from stress sensitivity to a depressive state: longitudinal twin study. *Br J Psychiatry* **195**(6): 498–503.

Winston, C., V. Maheshri, and F. Mannering. (2006). An exploration of the offset hypothesis using disaggregate data: the case of airbags and antilock brakes. *J Risk Uncertainty* **32**(2): 83–99.

Yusuf, S., S. Reddy, S. Ounpuu, and S. Anand. (2001). Global burden of cardiovascular diseases: part I: general considerations, the epidemiologic transition, risk factors, and impact of urbanization. *Circulation* **104**(22): 2746–2753.

5

Ubiquity and the Macrosocial Determinants of Population Health

WE HAVE THUS far surfaced three premises that lead to this chapter. First, we noted the health of populations is dependent ultimately on the health of the individuals within those populations, which is undoubtedly based on a cascade of factors that range from those that vary within populations to those that vary across populations. Second, we made the case that the factors that drive population health may vary across populations, and such factors may influence the overall shape and mean of distributions of population health. Third, we argued that for science to achieve the goal of improving the health of populations, we must focus our attention on those factors that are consequential and have the potential to matter most with regard to shifting the curve of population health. Given that shifting the curve is ultimately our goal as population health scientists, a focus on the factors that may indeed play such a role is a critical part of methodological scholarship in population health science.

This chapter builds on these premises to argue that many of the factors most central to the production of population health are macrosocial factors. By macrosocial factors we mean factors and systems above the level of organization of individuals that may shape population distributions of health and illness. They may include political structures and policies/laws, social network and migration patterns, economic indicators of structural wealth or disparity, culture and social norms, patterns of care access and preventive services, population density, and characteristics of the physical and social environment in which populations are embedded. There is a substantial and growing body of evidence that macrosocial factors are central drivers of population health

(Galea 2007) that shape the distributions of health within populations and predict variations in population health across populations. In this chapter we make the argument for the centrality of macrosocial factors in any scientific exercise around population health.

We build our argument in three sections. First, we describe the foundational principles that provide a framework for considering macrosocial factors. In particular, we focus on the ubiquity of macrosocial factors and how this has substantial health implications. Second, we provide examples of the macrosocial factors that have been a focus of the literature on population health, illustrating macrosocial thinking and how it has been applied across this discipline. The purpose of this section is to provide a flavor of how macrosocial determinants are assessed and included in population health science research. Third, we discuss some issues raised by the assessment of macrosocial factors in population health, and our role as population health scientists in the cross-disciplinary consideration of macrosocial drivers.

1.0 The Influence of Ubiquitous Exposures on Population Health

Factors that shape population health may be ubiquitous within the population—meaning, all individuals in the population are exposed. This has two implications for population health scientists. First, their very ubiquity makes it essential that we recognize macrosocial factors and consider how they may impact the health of populations affected by these factors, because small changes may translate to substantial public health implications. Second, however, their very ubiquity often makes it hard even to consider these factors, because the lack of variation within the population renders these factors difficult to observe.

This is effectively illustrated by considering an analogy. Let us consider goldfish in a bowl (Figure 5.1). The fish have a particular ecosystem that controls their temperature, toxin exposure, and chemical balance, and all the fish are exposed equally. To determine the "population" distribution of health in terms of the ecosystem of the bowl, we would need to compare across fishbowls. Suppose a fish population scientist observed that fish in one bowl were sicker than fish in another bowl. If she set about trying to understand this problem by looking only within the sick fishbowl to determine what makes some fish sick and some well, she misses the contribution of the ubiquitous factor—the water—that is different across bowls and accounts for fish

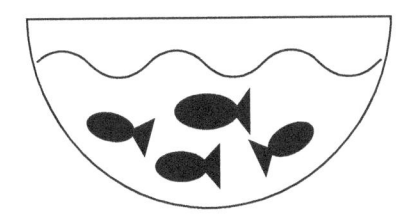

FIGURE 5.1 A metaphor for ubiquity. The goldfish are surrounded by water and everything they do is influenced by the quality of the water in which they live; therefore, water is a ubiquitous factor influencing the fish and needs to be taken into consideration every time we want to improve the lives of the fish.

sickness in one particular bowl. Therefore, if we compare risk factors between those who are sick and those who are not within the same bowl, we cannot discern the cause of the fish sickness. The cause of the sickness is the water in the bowl, but the fish cannot see the water as a potential cause because they are all exposed to it and surrounded by it.

Just like the water in the fishbowl, human populations face ubiquitous exposures that may have importance for public health. Like the fish, we share environmental characteristics such as air and the water supply. Depending on geography, we may also be exposed to living conditions, urbanicity, policies and laws, food supply, access to care, social networks, social norms, and a host of other factors at levels of organization broader than the individual and the individual's health behaviors. Collectively, we term these factors *macrosocial* because they are large in scale (macro) and often describe the ways in which we interact with each other and our environments (social). The ubiquity of these factors within environments and variance in these factors across environments makes them inextricable to discussions of what shapes population health. Macrosocial factors are systematic levers that create and maintain large-scale change, and even small changes to these ubiquitous causes can have a large impact on health at the population level.

Consider the following example. Income inequality has been associated with mortality across a wide variety of countries (Wilkinson and Pickett 2006, Kawachi and Subramanian 2014); countries with a larger gap between the very rich and the very poor in general have worse average health. Income inequality is a macrosocial factor; it is ubiquitous within each of the countries, and every member of the country is exposed to the income inequality of the country. Suppose we have a country with high-income inequality. We have a choice between investing resources in reducing exposure to a particularly harmful behavior that leads to mortality within the country (in our

POPULATION HEALTH SCIENCE

Table 5.1 Five-Year Mortality for Those Age 18 to 65 Years in a Country with High-Income Inequality

Drug Use Status	Died (n)	Alive (n)	Total (n)
Intravenous drug user	50	950	1000
Non-intravenous drug user	400	49,600	50,000
Total	450	50,550	51,000

example we will use intravenous drug use), or changing the distribution of wealth for the whole country.

Using the data presented in Table 5.1, we determine the number of intravenous (IV) drug users and non-IV drug users, and how many of these groups die during a 5-year period, and estimate the risk ratio and risk difference for the association between IV drug use and mortality:

$$\text{Risk Ratio} = \frac{\frac{50}{1,000}}{\frac{400}{50,000}} = 6.25$$

and

$$\text{Risk Difference} = \left(\frac{50}{1,000}\right) - \left(\frac{400}{50,000}\right) = 0.042.$$

In the country under study, the prevalence of IV drug use is 1.96% ((1,000/51,000) * 100) and IV drug users have 6.25 times the risk of mortality compared with non-IV drug users. For every 100 IV drug users, we expect 4.2 additional deaths in the age group of 18 to 65 years.

Now, let us consider the data if we reduce income inequality, specifying a modest association between income inequality and death. For the purpose of our example, we model a 1.25-fold increase in the risk of death associated with living in a highly unequal society. Imagine we reduce income inequality and obtain the data listed in Table 5.2.

Note that we kept the prevalence of IV drug use the same, at 1.96%, but we reduced deaths in each of the exposure groups by a factor of 1.25, commensurate with our reduction in income inequality. If we reorganize the data to compare the country before and after income inequality reduction (holding all else

Table 5.2 Five-Year Mortality for Those Age 18 to 65 Years after Reduction in Income Inequality

Drug Use Status	Died (n)	Alive (n)	Total (n)
Intravenous drug user	40	960	1000
Non-intravenous drug user	320	49,680	50,000
Total	360	50,640	51,000

constant), we obtain the data observed in Table 5.3. We then estimate the risk ratio (dividing the risk of mortality among IV drug users by the risk of mortality among the non-IV drug users) as well as the risk difference (subtracting the risk of mortality among non-IV drug users from the risk of mortality among IV drug users) to estimate the magnitude of the association between IV drug use and mortality.

$$\text{Risk Ratio} = \frac{\frac{450}{51,000}}{\frac{360}{51,000}} = 1.25$$

and

$$\text{Risk Difference} = \left(\frac{450}{51,000}\right) - \left(\frac{360}{51,000}\right) = 0.0018.$$

Thus, those in the unequal society have 1.25 times the risk of death and we expect 1.8 deaths per 1,000 persons exposed to the unequal society.

Comparing the magnitudes of effect between IV drug use and income inequality, we might assume IV drug use intervention may have more impact on mortality; the risk ratio is higher for IV drug use (6.25) than is the risk

Table 5.3 Comparison of 5-Year Mortality for Those Age 18 to 65 Years Before and after Change in Income Inequality

Timeline of Income Inequality	Died (n)	Alive (n)	Total (n)
Before change in income inequality	450	50,550	51,000
After change in income inequality	360	50,640	5,1000

> **BOX 5.1**
>
> **Fifth Foundational Principle of Population Health Science**
>
> Small changes in ubiquitous causes may result in more substantial change in the health of populations than larger changes in rarer causes.

ratio for income inequality (1.25); similarly, the risk difference for IV drug use is higher than the risk difference for income inequality. However, let us compare the actual number of lives affected. In the hypothetical income inequality intervention, we "saved" 90 lives (450 − 360 = 90). In our IV drug use example, we "save" an additional 4.2 times as many lives per 100 users; with 1000 total users in our population, we estimate that we save a maximum of 42 lives even if all IV drug users stopped using drugs.

Thus, we save more than twice the number of lives with the income inequality intervention than with an intervention for IV drug use that stops all users from using. This is because IV drug use is rare in the population whereas income inequality is ubiquitous. Although preventing harm associated with IV drug use is certainly an important goal for a healthy society, these results indicate we would achieve a greater overall good by reducing income inequality even though it is associated less with mortality than IV drug use.

This example illustrates a foundational principle of population health science (Box 5.1). In our example, we see that changing income inequality saves more lives than changing IV drug use.

2.0 Examples of Macrosocial Factors as Drivers of Population Health Distributions

In this section we discuss three examples to illustrate how macrosocial factors are central to the prediction of population health, but also difficult to measure and assess.

2.1 Macrosocial Determinants of Health Disparities in the United States

Blacks in the United States experience higher rates of morbidity and mortality than whites across multiple outcomes (Centers for Disease Control and

Prevention 2011). Disparities are present from birth; the risk of preterm delivery for black women is about twice that of whites (Rowley et al. 1993), and disparities in health continue throughout the life course. Although the United States has seen dramatic advancements in public health, racial disparities persist in life expectancy and in mortality from leading causes of death such as heart disease, hypertension, and diabetes (Winkleby et al. 1992, Mokdad et al. 2003, Centers for Disease Control and Prevention 2011, Olshansky et al. 2012). Known risk factors for poor health—including behavioral factors such as smoking and excessive alcohol consumption, as well as social factors such as chronic poverty—account only in part for racial disparities in health. Thus, research into additional factors that can explain these disparities remains a critical public health priority (Williams and Mohammed 2009, Centers for Disease Control and Prevention 2011), and substantial research has turned its attention to the way in which implicit biases and structural forms of discrimination—that is, the ubiquitous societal-level conditions that constrain individuals' opportunities, resources, and well-being based on race (Meyer 2003)—may affect health adversely.

The pervasive ways in which discrimination affects well-being have been documented extensively—from discrimination in the workforce (Bertrand and Mullainathan 2004) and in housing (Williams and Collins 2001, Keene and Geronimus 2011) to factors such as sentencing and incarceration for crimes (Uggen and Manza 2002, Alexander 2010). Growing evidence also indicates that exposure to systematic and structural forms of discrimination are associated with the development and persistence of chronic disease (Krieger 2012, Lukachko et al. 2014). For example, comparisons of mortality among whites and blacks in states with and without Jim Crow legislation in the decade between 1960 and 1970 have shown the highest mortality rates occurred in black populations within Jim Crow states and the lowest occurred among whites in these same states (Krieger 2012). Illustrating a population health science approach, researchers across disciplines have developed and tested theories for not only the overall effects of structural forms of discrimination, but also for the mechanisms through which these ubiquitous exposures may have an influence—from the "weathering" effects on cardiometabolic function to telomere length to epigenetic process, and to long-term effects on stress response pathways (Jackson and Knight 2006, Geronimus et al. 2010, Geronimus and Snow 2013). As such, these macrosocial factors, including policies and laws with historical legacies that remain central to the production of population health today, provide robust indicators of why health disparities emerge and how they predict variation in health at the population level differently between blacks and whites. Importantly, however, if we were to examine only what differentiates health outcomes among blacks in the United States, we may miss a major source of health that is ubiquitous in the environment: exposure to structural forms of discrimination.

2.2 Macrosocial Determinants of Alcohol-Related Consequences

An example of macrosocial drivers influencing population health distributions is seen in alcohol consumption and its related consequences. Alcohol consumption is part of the social fabric of many countries and has been for centuries. Although average per-capita consumption varies considerably across countries (Rehm et al. 2003, Rehm and Shield 2013), there is tremendous variability in alcohol consumption within countries. That is, within many countries, there is a portion of individuals who abstain, drink moderately, and drink heavily. The determinants of the shape of this distribution vary with respect to risk factors such as parental history of drinking, male sex, age, birth cohort, social networks and mixing, and many other factors. But, as is true in many population health indicators, the determinants of the mean alcohol consumption across countries are distinct from the causes of variation within the country.

This heterogeneity in mean alcohol consumption across countries reflects many factors, most notably the social norms around drinking and their variation across the world. Skog (1985) terms this mean variation "the collectivity of drinking cultures." Figure 5.2 is from a classic study conducted by Skog (1985), who demonstrated the distribution of alcohol consumption varies considerably across countries; those who are in the heaviest-drinking quartile in some countries would be categorized in the lightest-drinking quartile in other countries.

Thus, we may predict there are macrosocial determinants of alcohol consumption that can shift the distribution of consumption upward or downward overall without, perhaps, disturbing the standard deviation. In fact, there are many such examples of macrosocial determinants of alcohol consumption. A prominent example is alcohol taxation; a 2010 meta-analysis of more than 100 students with around 1,000 estimates indicated alcohol taxation reduces alcohol consumption at the population level, with about a 5% decrease in consumption for every 10% increase in alcohol taxes (Wagenaar et al. 2009). Alcohol taxes are an effective and cost-efficient way to reduce alcohol consumption in a population. Available evidence indicates drinkers across the

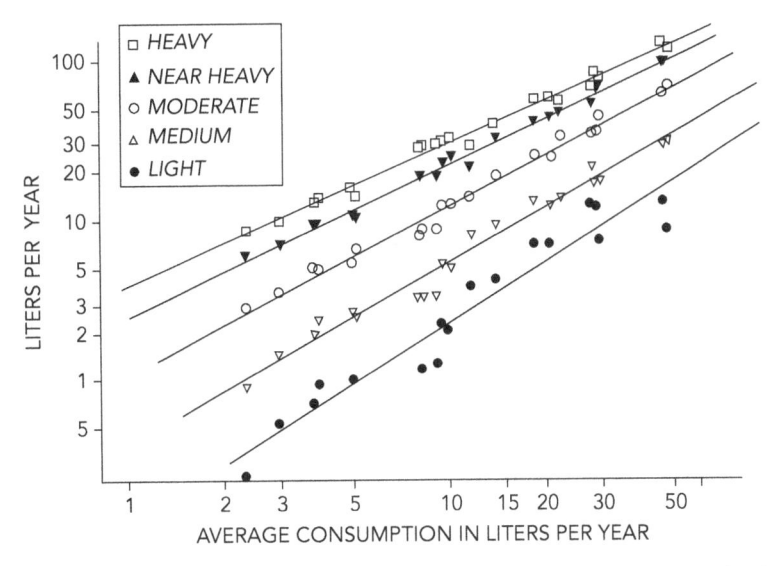

FIGURE 5.2 Relationship between average consumption and the consumption level of selected drinking groups (defined by percentiles) in 21 population surveys.
Note: The straight lines are least squares regressions. *Source*: Skog, O. J. (1985). The collectivity of drinking cultures: a theory of the distribution of alcohol consumption. *Br J Addict* 80(1): 90.

distribution of alcohol consumption are responsive to alcohol taxes (that is, both moderate and heavy drinkers, on average, drink less when taxes increase); thus, alcohol taxation is a classic example of a "curve-shifting" population health approach (Cook 1981, Cook and Tauchen 1982, Chaloupka et al. 2002, Wagenaar et al. 2009).

Furthermore, macrosocial determinants of population health are clearly apparent in determinants of harms from alcohol use at the population level. As shown in Figure 5.3, alcohol-associated motor vehicle crash fatalities have declined considerably during the past several decades, with substantial decreases throughout the 1980s and 1990s (Yi et al. 2006).

Although motor vehicle fatalities have been decreasing in the US population overall for decades (as a result of a combination of consumer protections such as safer vehicles, safety belts, air bags, and other macrosocial measures), alcohol-associated motor vehicle crashes in particular have benefited from a series of macrosocial measures (Room et al. 2005), including raising the minimum legal drinking age, reducing the legal blood alcohol content to drive, as well as more grassroots consumer campaigns such as Mothers Against Drunk Driving, which has not only advocated for legal policies around

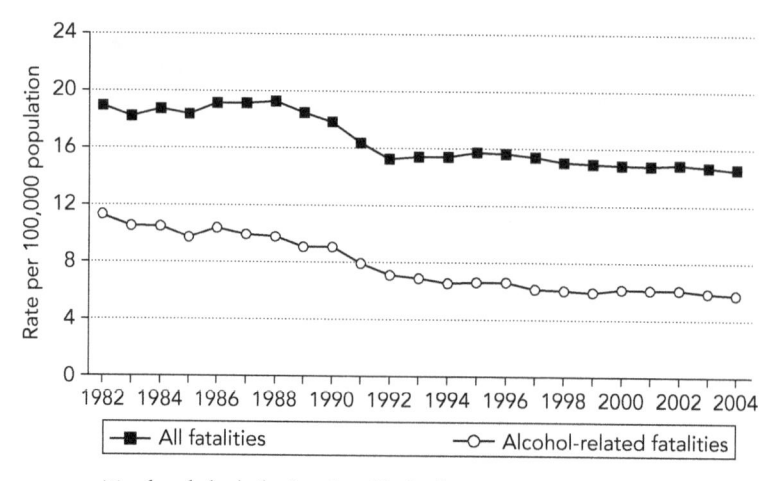

FIGURE 5.3 Total and alcohol-related traffic fatality rates per 100,000 population in the United States from 1982 to 2004.

Source: Yi, H., C. M. Chen, and G. D. Williams. (2006). *Surveillance report no. 76: trends in alcohol-related fatal traffic crashes, United States, 1982–2004*. Bethesda, MD: Division of Epidemiology and Prevention Research National Institute on Alcohol Abuse and Alcoholism.

alcohol-impaired drinking, but also has strived to change the social norm around driving drunk. Although "one for the road" was considered socially acceptable during the 1960s and 1970s, by the end of the 1980s, awareness of the harms associated with drunk driving and the ubiquity of messages to consider "designated drivers" changed the social landscape of bar and nightlife for drinkers.

2.3 Social Norms as Macrosocial Determinants: Unseen Yet Powerful Predictors of Population Health

An emerging area of research focuses on how social norms affect population health. Social norms refer generally to codes of conduct in ways of thinking and behaving. Theorists have called social norms the "grammar of social interaction" (Bicchieri 2006) because they provide an unspoken script regarding how to behave or think. Social norms have important social functions because they provide an efficient way to interact, a set of ground rules for behavior, and a set of sanctions when broken. Social norms thus maintain social order and provide a script for cooperation in social situations.

Social norms are pervasive in health behaviors, and an individual's perceptions of social norm are powerful predictors of engagement with various health-related factors, from tooth brushing to condom use to substance use.

For example, although alcohol consumption is legal for adults, there are social norms regarding the situations in which it is appropriate to drink, the amount that is appropriate to drink, and which beverages connote certain identities of the individuals consuming them (Greenfield and Room 1997). These norms maintain a social order with regard to alcohol consumption. The powerful salience of social norms can be seen in cigarette smoking (van den Putte et al. 2005, Scott et al. 2015). Although smoking was once a health behavior with limited sanctions, it is now increasingly considered an undesirable habit. Even in situations in which smoking is not legally sanctioned, it is now not normative for individuals to smoke in a variety of contexts that would have been considered socially acceptable previously (Karasek et al. 2012).

Social norms are difficult to study specifically because they are often unseen and pervasive. The ways in which social norms are expressed often derive from belief and expectation, as well prior knowledge and learned behavior. One way in which to visualize the impact of social norms is to capture population-level attitudes about health and health-related behavior. Empirical work has demonstrated, for example, that the proportion of adolescents who disapprove of alcohol and marijuana use varies substantially over time, and this variation predicts changes in the population-level prevalence of binge drinking and marijuana use (Keyes et al. 2011, 2012).

Social norms are tied to social identity in powerful ways that have pervasive impacts on behavior. Social identity can be conceived of as the set of norms and characteristics tied to a sense of who we are with respect to group membership (Tajfel and Turner 1979). Group membership provides a sense of belonging that creates an identity and, along with that identity, characteristics and health behaviors. For example, our social identities may be tied to geographic location (e.g., American, German, Brazilian), characteristics of us as people (e.g., woman, black, gay), occupation (e.g., doctor, musician, population health scientist), and defining life events (e.g., father, widow, earthquake survivor). This process helps us create meaning, but also establishes and enforces sets of social norms and, in some cases, can engender an us-versus-them mentality (Geronimus 2013). In fact, the associated stigma with belonging to certain groups has central implications for health and health behaviors, and is implicated in the development and persistence of health inequities across stigmatized groups (Phelan, Link et al. 2010, Link and Phelan 2014).

These social identities and the norms associated with them have meaning for many aspects of behavior and thoughts. For example, stereotype threat has been shown to be an important predictor of test performance. That is, individuals who, based on social identity, are generally stereotyped to be better or worse performers on a test will under- or overperform if they are asked to identify their social identity before the start of a test (Steele 1997). Blacks, for example, during experimental conditions perform worse on a test if they are asked to check a box with their self identified race before the start of a test. Women also underperform when asked to identify as women before a test, and Asian students overperform. Although test performance is not a health behavior per se, social norms and group membership have been demonstrated to affect factors such as alcohol and marijuana use (Ahern et al. 2008), mental health and cognitive coping mechanisms after stress (Wood and Parham 1990, Haley et al. 1996), and screening and preventive care (Suarez et al. 2000, Kinney et al. 2005, Williams and Jackson 2005).

3.0 The Implications of Macrosocial Determinants of Health for Population Health Science

Macrosocial determinants embed many of the population health indicators that continue to contribute to morbidity and mortality. Such effects are seen in examples such as alcohol consumption and related mortality, where there is wide variation in population means across countries, and macrosocial determinants such as taxation, policies, and social norms render population curve shifting across the distribution of consumption.

Because ubiquitous factors shape systems, delivery of care, norms, and the structures of exposures that become embedded in individual health decision making, they are core drivers of common complex disease in populations. They are, in fact, possibly *the* drivers of such disease in populations, although individual-level risk factors remain important components of population and public health as well. Conceptualization, assessment, and measurement of macrosocial forces that shape health are paramount to a research program that attends to the distribution and determinants of population health across time and geography.

A focus on ubiquitous causes thus has the potential to have a central impact on population health, and often drives distributions of population health. Yet, we often neglect or dismiss ubiquitous causes as not practical, feasible, or politically viable for change. Macrosocial determinants of health often involve structures and systems, such as political parties and policies, entrenched structural forms of discrimination and disenfranchisement, poverty and inequality, and other large-scale exposures with historical legacies. Considering how to change such factors is difficult, and, in a practical sense, changing such factors requires considerable capital. However, as population health scientists, a focus on macrosocial determinants is critical despite the challenges.

Change in macrosocial determinants of health is often not as intractable as we perhaps envision. For example, a robust body of literature indicates residential racial segregation is associated with a variety of adverse health indicators in the United States (Williams and Collins 2001, Krieger 2012). Residential segregation refers to the clustering of individuals in particular neighborhoods based on race, and national data indicate that many areas of the United States have high levels of segregation, in which individuals within any particular neighborhood are more likely to be similar racially than across neighborhoods. A population health science approach aims to understand the processes that generate racial segregation and the downstream mechanisms through which racial segregation generates adverse health indicators, and to evaluate the potential social and legal interventions that may impact such segregation. The challenge to this approach is, not infrequently, that it is too difficult to contemplate changing racial residential segregation. However, this is not really the case. There have been many ways in which residential segregation has been mitigated in the United States, such as restructuring the ways in which home loans are offered differentially across geographic locations, outlawing overt discrimination on the basis of race for renting or purchasing a home, creating more efficient means of transportation and commerce, and other broad policies and programs that intervene across levels of organization. At the core, it is important to remember that macrosocial factors are the result of deliberate actions we take as societies and, insofar as our job as population health scientists is to illustrate what drives health, we need to be unstinting in our focus on the factors that inevitably shape health and that can have enormous effects if manipulated. Social forces can act to change these factors as much as they acted to create them.

Regardless of whether there is a specific intervention, real or imagined, practical or impractical, that can be envisioned for the effects of macrosocial determinants on health, it remains within the purview of population health scientists to document the historical and current associations of such factors on health distributions in populations. Our charge is to explain patterns of health variation within and across populations. If macrosocial causes are important sources of variation, then their effects are important to document regardless of whether there is current potential for change in the exposure. Historical legacies of racism and racist policies, for example, are associated robustly with current health disparities (Krieger 2012). Although we cannot change the past, and there is no clear intervention on changing the effects of these historical legacies, is important to document and explain the fact that such legacies explain current distributions and patterns of health and mortality in the United States.

There is also a more subtle methodological point worth noting. In epidemiology and other quantitative health sciences, scholars pursuing the identification of causal effects have discussed how causal effects cannot be identified when exposures are not defined by the intervention with which they could be changed (VanderWeele and Robinson 2014). That is, unless there is a well-defined intervention for how an exposed person would become unexposed (Hernan and Taubman 2008, Glass et al. 2013), the assumptions that underlie the identification of the effect of that exposure on health are not met. This proposition has been met with controversy (Pearl 2009, Broadbent 2013, Glymour and Glymour 2014), especially among those advocating for the assessment of macrosocial determinants of health, wherein there are many potential interventions and thus many potential causal effects. While these debates remain under consideration, as population health scientists we should be specific about our exposures of interest, and thoughtful about the mechanisms through which they may impact health to construct clear, articulate comparisons to assess the impact of macrosocial determinants on population distributions of health.

4.0 Summary

Fifteen years ago, a set of papers in epidemiology asked the question: Should the mission of epidemiology be the eradication of poverty? (Rothman et al. 1998). Given that we know poverty is a fundamental cause of many of the health indicators and inequities we study, a natural question is whether we should be tasked with the goal of reducing these processes through large-scale and small-scale efforts. In this chapter we argue that quantitative population health science has no choice but to tackle poverty. The argument about the extent to which we should also be engaged in reducing it—and whether the same people who study it should also attempt to engage in work that seeks to transform society—remains. As population health scientists we need to examine systems and processes that are deeply embedded and multigenerational because they matter for health. The truth that macrosocial factors are difficult to mitigate makes it all the more incumbent that we interface in a cross-disciplinary way with researchers in political science, anthropology, biology, and sociology in ways that extend beyond simply identifying risk factors or correlates to truly meaningful process and mechanistic work.

The way in which we do this work and the questions we ask speak to our values and morals as scientists; to suggest our work is value free is fraught with error. Politics, power, and funding are real factors that shape the way in which our work is used, supported, and acted on, yet our job is to do good science, guided by values we acknowledge explicitly. We provide society with the options and the evidence for how to engage scientifically with the world and our health, and to analyze options for change that aspires to improve population health.

5.0 References

Ahern, J., S. Galea, A. Hubbard, L. Midanik, and S. L. Syme. (2008). 'Culture of drinking' and individual problems with alcohol use. *Am J Epidemiol* **167**(9): 1041–1049.

Alexander, M. (2010). *The new Jim Crow mass incarceration in the age of colorblindness.* New York: New Press.

Bertrand, M., and S. Mullainathan. (2004). Are Emily and Greg more employable than Lakisha and Jamal? A field experiment on labor market discrimination. *Am Econ Rev* **94**(4): 991–1013.

Bicchieri, C. (2006). *The grammar of society: the nature and dynamics of social norms.* New York: Cambridge University Press.

Broadbent, A. (2013). *Philosophy of epidemiology.* New York: Palgrave Macmillan.

Centers for Disease Control and Prevention. (2011). CDC health disparities and inequalities report: United States, 2011. *MMWR* **60**.

Chaloupka, F. J., M. Grossman, and H. Saffer. (2002). The effects of price on alcohol consumption and alcohol-related problems. *Alcohol Res Health* **26**(1): 22–34.

Cook, P. J. (1981). The effect of liquor taxes on drinking, cirrhosis, and auto accidents. In *Alcohol and public policy: Beyond the shadow of prohibition.* M. H. Moore and D. R. Gerstein, editors. Washington, DC: National Academy Press: 255–285.

Cook, P. J., and G. Tauchen. (1982). The effect of taxes on heavy drinking. *Bell J Econ* **13**(2): 379–390.

Galea, S. (2007). *Macrosocial determinants of population health.* New York: Springer.

Geronimus, A. T. (2013). Jedi public health: Leveraging contingencies of social identity to grasp and eliminate racial health inequality. In *Mapping 'race': Critical approaches to health disparities research.* L. E. Gomez and N. Lopez, editors. New Brunswick, NJ: Rutgers University Press: 163–178.

Geronimus, A. T., M. T. Hicken, J. A. Pearson, S. J. Seashols, K. L. Brown, and T. D. Cruz. (2010). Do US black women experience stress-related accelerated biological aging? A novel theory and first population-based test of black–white differences in telomere length. *Hum Nat* **21**(1): 19–38.

Geronimus, A. T., and R. C. Snow. (2013). The mutability of women's health with age: the sometimes rapid, and often enduring, health consequences of injustice. In

Women & health. M. Goldman, K. Rexrode, and R. Troisi, editors. Salt Lake City, UT: Academic Press: 21–32.

Glass, T. A., S. N. Goodman, M. A. Hernan, and J. M. Samet. (2013). Causal inference in public health. *Annu Rev Public Health* **34**: 61–75.

Glymour, C., and M. R. Glymour. (2014). Commentary: race and sex are causes. *Epidemiology* **25**(4): 488–490.

Greenfield, T. K., and R. Room. (1997). Situational norms for drinking and drunkenness: trends in the US adult population, 1979–1990. *Addiction* **92**(1): 33–47.

Haley, W. E., D. L. Roth, M. I. Coleton, G. R. Ford, C. A. West, R. P. Collins, et al. (1996). Appraisal, coping, and social support as mediators of well-being in black and white family caregivers of patients with Alzheimer's disease. *J Consult Clin Psychol* **64**(1): 121–129.

Hernan, M. A., and S. L. Taubman. (2008). Does obesity shorten life? The importance of well-defined interventions to answer causal questions. *Int J Obes (Lond)* **32**(Suppl 3): S8–S14.

Jackson, J. S., and K. M. Knight. (2006). Race and self-regulatory health behaviors: the role of the stress response and the HPA axis in physical and mental health disparities. In *Social structures, aging, and self-regulation in the elderly.* K. W. Schaie and L. Carstensen, editors. New York: Springer: 189–209.

Karasek, D., J. Ahern, and S. Galea. (2012). Social norms, collective efficacy, and smoking cessation in urban neighborhoods. *Am J Public Health* **102**(2): 343–351.

Kawachi, I., and S. Subramanian. (2014). Income inequality. In *Social epidemiology.* L. Berkman, I. Kawachi, and M. Glymour, editors. New York: Oxford University Press: 126–152.

Keene, D. E., and A. T. Geronimus. (2011). 'Weathering' HOPE VI: the importance of evaluating the population health impact of public housing demolition and displacement. *J Urban Health* **88**(3): 417–435.

Keyes, K. M., J. E. Schulenberg, P. M. O'Malley, L. D. Johnston, J. G. Bachman, G. Li, et al. (2011). The social norms of birth cohorts and adolescent marijuana use in the United States, 1976–2007. *Addiction* **106**(10): 1790–1800.

Keyes, K. M., J. E. Schulenberg, P. M. O'Malley, L. D. Johnston, J. G. Bachman, G. Li, et al. (2012). Birth cohort effects on adolescent alcohol use: the influence of social norms from 1976 to 2007. *Arch Gen Psychiatry* **69**(12): 1304–1313.

Kinney, A. Y., L. E. Bloor, C. Martin, and R. S. Sandler. (2005). Social ties and colorectal cancer screening among blacks and whites in North Carolina. *Cancer Epidemiol Biomarkers Prev* **14**(1): 182–189.

Krieger, N. (2012). Methods for the scientific study of discrimination and health: an ecosocial approach. *Am J Public Health* **102**(5): 936–944.

Link, B. G., and J. Phelan. (2014). Stigma power. *Soc Sci Med* **103**: 24–32.

Lukachko, A., M. L. Hatzenbuehler, and K. M. Keyes. (2014). Structural racism and myocardial infarction in the United States. *Soc Sci Med* **103**: 42–50.

Meyer, I. H. (2003). Prejudice as stress: conceptual and measurement problems. *Am J Public Health* **93**(2): 262–265.

Mokdad, A. H., E. S. Ford, B. A. Bowman, W. H. Dietz, F. Vinicor, V. S. Bales, et al. (2003). Prevalence of obesity, diabetes, and obesity-related health risk factors, 2001. *JAMA* **289**(1): 76–79.

Olshansky, S. J., T. Antonucci, L. Berkman, R. H. Binstock, A. Boersch-Supan, J. T. Cacioppo, et al. (2012). Differences in life expectancy due to race and educational differences are widening, and many may not catch up. *Health Aff (Millwood)* **31**(8): 1803–1813.

Pearl, J. (2009). Causal inference in statistics: an overview. *Statistics Survey* **3**: 96–146.

Phelan, J. C., B. G. Link, and P. Tehranifar. (2010). Social conditions as fundamental causes of health inequalities: theory, evidence, and policy implications. *J Health Soc Behav* **51**(Suppl): S28–S40.

Rehm, J., N. Rehm, R. Room, M. Monteiro, G. Gmel, D. Jernigan, et al. (2003). The global distribution of average volume of alcohol consumption and patterns of drinking. *Eur Addict Res* **9**(4): 147–156.

Rehm, J., and K. D. Shield. (2013). Global alcohol-attributable deaths from cancer, liver cirrhosis, and injury in 2010. *Alcohol Res* **35**(2): 174–183.

Room, R., T. Babor, and J. Rehm. (2005). Alcohol and public health. *Lancet* **365**(9458): 519–530.

Rothman, K. J., H. O. Adami, and D. Trichopoulos. (1998). Should the mission of epidemiology include the eradication of poverty? *Lancet* **352**(9130): 810–813.

Rowley, D. L., C. J. Hogue, C. A. Blackmore, C. D. Ferre, K. Hatfield-Timajchy, P. Branch, et al. (1993). Preterm delivery among African-American women: a research strategy. *Am J Prev Med* **9**(6 Suppl): 1–6.

Scott, K. A., M. J. Mason, and J. D. Mason. (2015). I'm not a smoker: Constructing protected prototypes for risk behavior. *J Bus Res* **68**(10): 2198–2206.

Skog, O. J. (1985). The collectivity of drinking cultures: a theory of the distribution of alcohol consumption. *Br J Addict* **80**(1): 83–99.

Steele, C. M. (1997). A threat in the air: how stereotypes shape intellectual identity and performance. *Am Psychol* **52**(6): 613–629.

Suarez, L., A. G. Ramirez, R. Villarreal, J. Marti, A. McAlister, G. A. Talavera, et al. (2000). Social networks and cancer screening in four US Hispanic groups. *Am J Prev Med* **19**(1): 47–52.

Tajfel, H., and J. C. Turner. (1979). An integrative theory of intergroup conflict. In *The social psychology of intergroup relations*. W. G. Austin and S. Worchel, editors. Monterey, CA: Brooks-Cole Publishing: 33–47.

Uggen, C., and J. Manza. (2002). Demographic contraction? Political consequences of felon disenfranchisement in the United States. *Am Soc Rev* **67**(6): 777–803.

van den Putte, B., M. C. Yzer, and S. Brunsting. (2005). Social influences on smoking cessation: a comparison of the effect of six social influence variables. *Prev Med* **41**(1): 186–193.

VanderWeele, T. J., and W. R. Robinson. (2014). On the causal interpretation of race in regressions adjusting for confounding and mediating variables. *Epidemiology* **25**(4): 473–484.

Wagenaar, A. C., M. J. Salois, and K. A. Komro. (2009). Effects of beverage alcohol price and tax levels on drinking: a meta-analysis of 1003 estimates from 112 studies. *Addiction* **104**(2): 179–190.

Wilkinson, R. G., and K. E. Pickett. (2006). Income inequality and population health: a review and explanation of the evidence. *Soc Sci Med* **62**(7): 1768–1784.

Williams, D. R., and C. Collins. (2001). Racial residential segregation: a fundamental cause of racial disparities in health. *Public Health Rep* **116**(5): 404–416.

Williams, D. R., and P. B. Jackson. (2005). Social sources of racial disparities in health. *Health Aff (Millwood)* **24**(2): 325–334.

Williams, D. R., and S. A. Mohammed. (2009). Discrimination and racial disparities in health: evidence and needed research. *J Behav Med* **32**(1): 20–47.

Winkleby, M. A., D. E. Jatulis, E. Frank, and S. P. Fortmann. (1992). Socioeconomic status and health: how education, income, and occupation contribute to risk factors for cardiovascular disease. *Am J Public Health* **82**(6): 816–820.

Wood, J. B., and I. A. Parham. (1990). Coping with perceived burden: ethnic and cultural issues in Alzheimer's family caregiving. *J Appl Gerontol* **9**(3): 325–339.

Yi, H., C. M. Chen, and G. D. Williams. (2006). *Surveillance report no. 76: trends in alcohol-related fatal traffic crashes: United States, 1982–2004*. Bethesda, MD: Division of Epidemiology and Prevention Research National Institute on Alcohol Abuse and Alcoholism.

6

Causal Architecture to Understand What Matters Most

THEORY

THUS FAR IN this text we have explored the foundations of population health science with a focus on understanding how to conceptualize the causes of population health. We have done so with a very particular goal in mind. Our aim is to create a structure for the field in how we approach research questions with a lens toward producing consequential results that improve the health of populations. We advocate conceptual thinking that grounds itself in macro-social causes; shifting the curve of population health; examining measures of association that are not just strong in magnitude and statistical significance, but also in meaningfulness; and clarifying our thinking through the lens of consequential approaches to population health science (Galea 2013). Our aim in this clarification is to suggest a critical view through which we invest our intellectual and material resources. Part of this critical view involves examining the dominant paradigms in research and science that currently hold weight in the field, and thinking about how we might adapt these paradigms in important ways to push the field toward a science that sets as its center the idea we pursue relentlessly public health questions of consequence.

Therefore, we now move on, in the next three chapters, to grapple with how we can best use this understanding to guide our focus in population health.

Note: Portions of the text in this chapter are adapted from Keyes, K. M., and S. Galea. (2015). "What matters most: quantifying an epidemiology of consequence." *Ann Epidemiol* **25**, 305–311.

First, in the next two chapters, we build on current approaches in epidemiology toward articulating an approach that embeds a consequentialist approach toward population health science. In the first of these chapters we discuss a traditional risk factor approach to studying disease, and some limitations for that approach for population health science. In the second chapter we provide some quantitative examples that can help reorient our research questions with a framework that aligns more closely with the values of population health science we advocate in this book. In the subsequent chapter we ask how we may value population health approaches more generally, and preventive efforts specifically.

1.0 The Limits of Risk Factor Approaches to the Study of Disease

The science of public health often reports series of exposures correlated with health indicators of interest, termed *risk factors*. In the pantheon of epidemiological literature, studies are reported often with conflicting results. For example, there remains debate regarding the health consequences of being overweight (Lewis et al. 2009, Berrington de Gonzalez et al. 2010, Flegal and Kalantar-Zadeh 2013), the effects of specific dietary foods such as berries (Sesso et al. 2007, Cassidy et al. 2013), butter (Kromhout et al. 2011, Holmberg and Thelin 2013, Chowdhury et al. 2014), salt (Bayer et al. 2012, Johns et al. 2013), and alcohol (Keyes and Miech 2013) on health, as well as purported health-sustaining supplements such as multivitamins (Guallar et al. 2013).

Risk factor epidemiology has been the dominant analytic paradigm to identify causes of disease for several decades. Although conceptual approaches such as social and life course epidemiology have broadened our understanding substantially of the factors we may consider to be "causes" of disease and illness (Kuh et al. 2003, Berkman and Kawachi 2014), the common risk factor approach has remained one in which we use ever-more sophisticated analytic methods to identify causes that increase the risk of a particular pathology. Although this approach has proved useful and has met with considerable successes (Centers for Disease and Prevention 2011), the past 30 years of risk factor epidemiology has also presented us with a baffling and almost endless array of potentially causal observations.

The search for modifiable risk factors that prevent the onset of chronic disease is important and worthy of our time, effort, and resources. There is nothing inherently inefficient with the discipline producing a long list of risk factors, and it is the nature of scientific inquiry to articulate arguments both for and against particular observations (Greenland et al. 2004). We collect data, present findings, question them, refine hypotheses, incorporate refuting evidence, and move our understanding forward slowly and systematically until new data, new hypotheses, and new knowledge from across disciplines and designs upend our previously held paradigms (Popper 1935). Increasingly, causal models have been applied within epidemiology, improved on, refined, and expanded to allow researchers to provide more precise estimates of "causal effects" of a single risk factor on a health outcome (Robins et al. 2000, Petersen et al. 2006, VanderWeele and Hernan 2013, Gatto et al. 2014).

Because the field of risk factors is relatively well mined and we have a set of "usual suspects" (smoking, diet, poverty, toxins), we attempt to refine and reframe the extent to which previously identified associations are causal with increasingly restrictive samples, large sample sizes, and precise and methodologically sophisticated analyses to control for confounding and other sources of potential internal validity bias. This is entirely reasonable if the goal is to isolate the causal effect of an exposure on an outcome. However, more work needs to be done after causal identification if our overall goal is to improve population health, and if those in the sample for causal identification are not representative of the population in which we would like to intervene. In the latter case, we may have difficulty assessing the extent to which the exposure causes disease in our particular population, given its distributions of other causes of the disease, as we shall discuss later in this chapter.

The natural consequence of a risk factor approach focused on individual-level associations is the current era of predictive and personalized preventive medicine (Smith 2011, Ramos et al. 2012). If we have a set of 20 risk factors, each soaking up some small amount of variance, it becomes an almost natural next step to create predictive equations from them to identify the risks associated with individuals rather than populations. In fact, predictive medicine is now being recommended as a potential use of epidemiological data across several disciplines (Hood and Flores 2012, Li et al. 2015). The basic mathematical limitations of predictive equations for understanding, much less intervening in, population health have been well documented (Pepe et al. 2004, Keyes et al. 2015), and the utility of such models for public health is questionable (Krieger 2011, Smith 2011). We review the limits of predictive medicine for population health in more detail in Chapter 10.

Therefore, our risk factor-based value system can, based on the inputs we give and the questions we ask, detract from the goal of improving population health. Charged with conducting comparative work that can guide impact (e.g., What can we do that would improve the health of the population the most?), we often find ourselves focusing on better estimating the causal effects of single exposures (e.g., Did X cause Y?). Although the question "Did X cause Y?" is fundamental to science, as population health scientists we must be guided by whether we are asking about the right Xs, whether it matters that X caused Y without knowing about the context and co-occurring causes around X, and whether trial after trial of increasingly precise estimation of Xs is of real relevance.

Thus, risk factor approaches can, in some circumstances, trap us in a paradigm that Rockhill (2005) called "the increasingly reductionist hunt for causes." Rockhill (2005) and others (Shy 1997, Pepe et al. 2004, Wacholder 2005) suggest that most causal effects, even if they are relatively large, have little discriminatory ability at the individual level (which is why predictive medicine for complex chronic disease prevention faces serious challenges), and that a focus on shaping population health requires a movement away from the hunting for individual-level single causes of disease toward a more population health-oriented framework that acknowledges as paramount our interest in the distribution of potential causes at the population level (Rose 1985, Maldonado and Greenland 2002, Ahern et al. 2008, Poole 2010, Xie 2013).

The debate over the efficiency of risk factor approaches within the framework of our charge as population health scientists has raged for more than two decades. In his presidential address to the Society for Epidemiologic Research in 1993, for example, Milton Terris (1993) challenged the field by noting the following:

> We cannot remain indefinitely in our ivory towers; they may crumble around us. We need to foster epidemiologic research, not only by improving our methodology and sharing our scientific experience, but by helping to convince the American public and its legislators that prevention is far more important than treatment, that our expanded agenda for research needs full legislative and financial support, and that the application of our findings to improve the health of the public must become the highest priority for health policy in the United States. (p. 146)

Terris has certainly not been alone in calling to action a focus on translation and implementation of our science for public health improvement (Shy 1997, Rockhill 2005, McKeown 2009, Krieger 2012, Kuller 2013). Of course, few would argue against a focus on research questions that have direct and demonstrable ability to shift the curve of population health. After the relatively "low-hanging fruit" of factors such as cigarette smoking served as the benchmark through which modern epidemiological methods were developed (Morabia 2014), the risk factor approach has been reproduced and reified for relatively small effects and less stable science (Taubes 1995).

2.0 Population Health Science Approach to Studying Causes by Focusing on What Matters Most

The emphasis on identifying risk factors within a paradigm that hunts for precise causal effects obscures what we argue is the broader goal of the field of population health science—an attempt to identify what matters most. This approach urges us to identify what we can do about those factors that do indeed matter most for the health of populations, which necessarily involves both theory-driven approaches and a pragmatic assessment of what is likely to make a difference. Instrumentally, we focus on the relative weight of risk factors in producing poor health within and across populations.

An approach to understanding what matters most must rely inevitably on theory, hypothesis, and data-driven assessments of the multifactorial causal structures that produce population health, must acknowledge that single causes do not act in isolation, and must believe that understanding the nature of disease requires comprehending the broader network of causal structures (Krieger 1994, Marshall and Galea 2015). Such an approach requires us to model and test such structures, focusing less on the individual effects of exposures that penetrate the model, and instead explicate which factors—from the ubiquitous to the rare—are likely to have a large population impact. We must then narrow in on creative designs and broad comparisons to assess the public health impact of these factors as well as the factors for which they interact.

We do not intend to suggest that research on rare exposures and rare disease should be abandoned; such research is critical to scientific insight. For example, vaginal tumors are quite rare, but the discovery that in utero DES exposure is linked causally to the emergence of tumors at an early age was a breakthrough in our understanding of carcinogenesis (Herbst et al. 1971).

How, then, do we go about the practice of assessing the impact of potentially causal factors on outcomes that matter? We advocate for explicit focus on the prevalence of the factor, the prevailing hypothesized causes that interact with the factor, the causal structure that underlies the factor, as well as the prevalence of the health condition under study; all of these determine what is consequential for public health. Foundationally, we know that what matters most are factors that are going to affect the population on a large scale. And we also know that factors that will affect the population on a large scale are those that have very big effects and/or are very prevalent (Pepe et al. 2004, Rockhill 2005). A more rigorous focus on the absolute change in population health associated with exposures of interest has captured the attention of the methodological literature (Poole 2010, VanderWeele and Hernan 2013), and several measures and indices produced by the field during the past several decades have been build from solid risk factor methodological tools (Wacholder 2005). We provide further quantitative detail on such an approach in Chapter 7; here we describe a general conceptual approach to such investigations focused on assessing causal architecture.

3.0 An Approach Focused on Causal Architecture

Consider, for example, the basic directed acyclic graph for an exposure E and its potential causal relation with an outcome D. E and D share a set of antecedent causes Z. The current dominant approach to epidemiological inquiry is to determine whether E is independent of D conditional on all Zs. Scenarios become more complicated with time-varying covariates and more complicated structures, but in the end we often endeavor to determine whether E is independent of D. Rather than this traditional approach, however, let us consider an approach that assesses the causal architecture around E. Using such an approach, we acknowledge, assess, and model not just the complex structure that surrounds the association between single exposures and outcomes, but also the underlying architecture that activates these exposures. Disease is then located explicitly in a set of co-occurring causes. If, indeed, our goal is to understand the natural history of the health indicators that matter most in our populations, and our goal is to elucidate the universality of disease processes to advance scientific inquiry, such an approach is required. Causal architecture requires creativity, acknowledgment of the unknown, and comfort living in the ambiguity of stitching together causal stories rather than, or in addition to, imperfect estimations of causal effects that may or may not be meaningful, depending on the prevalence of co-occurring causes.

In Figure 6.1 we provide a comparison between types of questions that we ask using the traditional approach versus the causal architecture approach. Our traditional epidemiological technique is to ask: Is exposure associated with disease? Is exposure associated with disease controlling for a set of confounders? Does exposure interact with any factors to produce disease? What are the mechanisms through which exposure works? We have a well defined and increasingly sophisticated set of methods for addressing each of these questions, although sophistication and elegance of our modeling approaches

Traditional Risk Factor Approach	Causal Architecture
Is E associated with D? Is E associated with D controlling for a set of confounders? Does E interact with any factors to produce D? What are the mechanisms through which E works?	What is the structure of causes that underlie D? Do these causes work together or separately? Which causes are the most prevalent in the population for which we want to improve public health?

FIGURE 6.1 Traditional risk factor approaches versus causal architecture: how we can ask population health science questions differently.

alone are no match for the creativity and ingenuity of the researcher who is programming them (Cartwright 1999). A causal architecture approach, on the other hand, asks: What is the structure of causes that underlie disease? Do these causes work together or separately? And, most important, which causes are the most prevalent in the population for which we want to improve public health? This is an alternative framing and recalibration of our goals and our objectives as population health practitioners.

One clear example of such a causal architecture approach could be applied to the study of obesity, an outcome with clear public health relevance and a plethora of identified risk factors. There has been tremendous interest in identifying genetic underpinnings of obesity, and a great deal of effort committed to quantifying the effect of gene variants such as *FTO* on risk for obesity as well as explaining population variance in obesity risk (Peng et al. 2011, Park et al. 2013, Warrington et al. 2015). Yet we suggest this is perhaps too narrow a question, given that the social, political, and topographic environment is critical to obesity risk. In fact, emerging evidence indicates phenomena such as cohort of birth modify the effect of the *FTO* gene (Rosenquist et al. 2015), suggesting that the social structures in which we are embedded and develop shape the way in which molecular markers influence our health. Further expansion on the way in which risks for obesity are distributed across populations, interact with each other in dynamic ways, and spread across networks of individuals underlies a causal architecture approach and forces us to creatively prepare data and construct designs that articulate the broader structure in which obesity and its related health indicators are embedded.

4.0 Implications for Population Health Science

It is hard to argue that we should not be thinking about what matters most as we endeavor to build our research questions and design studies to answer these questions. The next question, then, is: How do we identify what matters most?

We suggest there are four key factors that we need to grapple with as a discipline as we move toward aligning population health science as a rigorous discipline with specific foundational principles. First, we need to move beyond a risk factor approach, in which the effects of exposures on outcomes are estimated, to a causal architecture approach, in which the causal structure that underlies our exposures and outcomes is hypothesized fully. In this way, we can be more attentive to ubiquitous exposures with the potential for intervention, to the way in which interactions among exposures may drive high-risk groups, and to the way in which dynamic contexts within and across populations may influence causal pathways. Although prevalent exposures are just one part of a dynamic inquiry that shapes priorities for population health sciences, we suggest that such considerations be brought to the fore in a more prominent way, and that an emphasis on how research can translate into shifting population health may aid in the prioritization of potential research and action avenues.

Second, engaging critically in what matters most for population health suggests almost inevitably that we are going to be increasing assessments of upstream causes prevalent in early-life, such as material deprivation, early-childhood education, and child adversity. These are not easy to change, and some argue it is not in our purview to change them (Rothman et al. 1998), as mentioned in Chapter 5. However, disciplines across the social and economic sciences are increasingly forming a consensus that these early-life and macro-policy-related factors are the critical drivers of many adult outcomes, including social and economic well-being and cognitive ability (Ludwig and Phillips 2008, McLaughlin et al. 2012, Heckman and Mosso 2014, Huang et al. 2014). Consider the case of exposure to crack cocaine and offspring health. Although the crack epidemic of the 1980s led to many sensational news stories about the health of offspring born to mothers addicted to crack cocaine, a long-term follow-up of children born to crack-addicted women, to nonaddicted women in the same social class, and to a control group of women found there was little effect of crack exposure on any cognitive or behavioral outcome assessed (Betancourt, Yang et al. 2011), but there was a substantial effect of poverty.

Those children born in deprived conditions, regardless of whether the mother used crack during pregnancy, were at a long-term disadvantage on almost every outcome measured. This underscores the what-matters-most approach: based on these data, what matters for ability and achievement is overcoming deprivation, and enhancing resources and support for families living in poverty. An emphasis on understanding and mitigating the effects of childhood poverty throughout the life course is, thus, arguably more important for public health than mitigating in utero exposures to substances. Although resources for pregnant women who are using substances should undoubtedly be allocated to achieving and maintaining sobriety, a focus on prenatal substance use is, perhaps, missing what matters most for long-term offspring health.

Third, internal validity of our studies to estimate precise causal effects is critical, and innovative tools continue to be generated across many disciplines (Munoz and van der Laan 2012, Keil et al. 2014, Naimi et al. 2014, Westreich 2014, Naimi and Kaufman 2015). Although internal validity is central to the conduct of science, there are and have always been concerns about generalizability beyond the study sample from tightly controlled experiments and analyses of specific subgroups chosen for comparability of groups (Greenhouse et al. 2008, Dekkers et al. 2010, Hernan and VanderWeele 2011). If we are concerned about what matters most for population health, however, generalizability and external validity become more prominent concerns as we endeavor to understand the distributions of risk factors and causal exposures that reside in the specific contexts in the populations we aim to study. As such, an elevation of external validity and representativeness of samples forces us to be concerned about the facts emerging from our studies and the extent to which they are providing insights that apply to large populations (Keyes and Galea 2014). Such concerns inevitably center on external validity. A causal architecture approach aids in this endeavor by promoting the application of theoretical models that take into account explicitly the prevalence and distributions of causes as well as their interactions. For example, although replication of study findings increases our confidence in their validity, nonreplication may be telling us something crucial about causal architecture across populations.

Fourth, a cornerstone of shifting paradigms within any discipline is education of up-and-coming scholars. Shifts in goals and framing of a discipline can be gradual and subtle, but they inevitably land at the feet of younger generations of scientists to proliferate and innovate. This is not to suggest that current and previous generations of scholars within our discipline have not been at the forefront of calls for recalibration of our thinking on the meaning and impact of population health science; however, a critical self-reflection on how we train and socialize scholars to focus on what matters most will be paramount to enacting an approach that focuses attention on curve shifting in population health. These concerns are, in part, what motivated the writing of this book; we the hope to challenge scholars to engage with us in these questions about quantification of population health science initiatives.

As we articulated in early chapters of this text, Geoffrey Rose's seminal contributions to defining population science have formed many vertebrae in the backbone of our understanding of how to influence public health (Rose 1985, Rose et al. 2008). Rose illuminated the foundational methodological principle that those factors that contribute to variation within a population may differ from the factors that contribute to variation in incidence across populations. When we conceptualize research agendas and craft public health responses to health problems, we must not lose sight of the fact that causes may be ubiquitous in one context, and therefore invariant, yet may still drive the health of society. Within this framework stands the current state of epidemiological research. Much has been written about paradigms of science (Fleck 1981, Kuhn 1981), and in epidemiology, the past 40 years have heralded the era of the risk factor, understanding and isolating insufficient and unnecessary—yet hopefully important—causes of complex health indicators. However, the potential for new risk factor discovery has yielded few novel insights of late, underscoring a call for new directions in the discipline, including integration of risk factor epidemiology with a broader platform of ecological and environmental assessments (Krieger 2012, Coughlin 2014), movement away from so-called "black box" epidemiology to illuminating the mechanisms through which risk factors operate (Petersen et al. 2006, Nandi et al. 2014, VanderWeele 2014), and integration of epidemiological principles with broader attempts to mine increasingly available biological and clinical data at the population level (Hood and Flores 2012). A what-matters-most lens has the potential to clarify our thinking, focus our scholarship, and help guide our pedagogical focus toward preparing the next generation of scientists to engage with a population health science of consequence.

5.0 References

Ahern, J., M. R. Jones, E. Bakshis, and S. Galea. (2008). Revisiting Rose: comparing the benefits and costs of population-wide and targeted interventions. *Milbank Q* 86(4): 581–600.

Bayer, R., D. M. Johns, and S. Galea. (2012). Salt and public health: contested science and the challenge of evidence-based decision making. *Health Aff (Millwood)* 31(12): 2738–2746.

Berkman, L. F., and I. O. Kawachi. (2014). *Social epidemiology.* Oxford: Oxford University Press.

Berrington de Gonzalez, A., P. Hartge, J. R. Cerhan, A. J. Flint, L. Hannan, R. J. MacInnis, et al. (2010). Body-mass index and mortality among 1.46 million white adults. *N Engl J Med* 363(23): 2211–2219.

Betancourt, L. M., W. Yang, N. L. Brodsky, P. R. Gallagher, E. K. Malmud, J. M. Giannetta, et al. (2011). Adolescents with and without gestational cocaine exposure: longitudinal analysis of inhibitory control, memory and receptive language. *Neurotoxicol Teratol* 33(1): 36–46.

Cartwright, N. (1999). *The dappled world: a study of the boundaries of science.* Cambridge: Cambridge University Press.

Cassidy, A., K. J. Mukamal, L. Liu, M. Franz, A. H. Eliassen, and E. B. Rimm. (2013). High anthocyanin intake is associated with a reduced risk of myocardial infarction in young and middle-aged women. *Circulation* 127(2): 188–196.

Centers for Disease Control and Prevention. (2011). Ten great public health achievements: United States, 2001–2010. *MMWR Morb Mortal Wkly Rep* 60(19): 619–623.

Chowdhury, R., S. Warnakula, S. Kunutsor, F. Crowe, H. A. Ward, L. Johnson, et al. (2014). Association of dietary, circulating, and supplement fatty acids with coronary risk: a systematic review and meta-analysis. *Ann Intern Med* 160(6): 398–406.

Coughlin, S. S. (2014). Toward a road map for global-omics: a primer on -omic technologies. *Am J Epidemiol* 180(12): 1188–1195.

Dekkers, O. M., E. von Elm, A. Algra, J. A. Romijn, and J. P. Vandenbroucke. (2010). How to assess the external validity of therapeutic trials: a conceptual approach. *Int J Epidemiol* 39(1): 89–94.

Fleck, L. (1981). *Genesis and development of a scientific fact.* Chicago: Chicago University Press.

Flegal, K. M., and K. Kalantar-Zadeh. (2013). Overweight, mortality and survival. *Obesity (Silver Spring)* 21(9): 1744–1745.

Galea, S. (2013). An argument for a consequentialist epidemiology. *Am J Epidemiol* 178(8): 1185–1191.

Gatto, N. M., U. B. Campbell, and S. Schwartz. (2014). An organizational schema for epidemiologic causal effects. *Epidemiology* 25(1): 88–97.

Greenhouse, J. B., E. E. Kaizar, K. Kelleher, H. Seltman, and W. Gardner. (2008). Generalizing from clinical trial data: a case study: the risk of suicidality among pediatric antidepressant users. *Stat Med* 27(11): 1801–1813.

Greenland, S., M. Gago-Dominguez, and J. E. Castelao. (2004). The value of risk-factor ('black-box') epidemiology. *Epidemiology* 15(5): 529–535.

Guallar, E., S. Stranges, C. Mulrow, L. J. Appel, and E. R. Miller, III. (2013). Enough is enough: stop wasting money on vitamin and mineral supplements. *Ann Intern Med* 159(12): 850–851.

Heckman, J. J., and S. Mosso. (2014). The economics of human development and social mobility. *Annu Rev Econom* 6: 689–733.

Herbst, A. L., H. Ulfelder, and D. C. Poskanzer. (1971). Adenocarcinoma of the vagina: association of maternal stilbestrol therapy with tumor appearance in young women. *N Engl J Med* **284**(15): 878–881.

Hernan, M. A., and T. J. VanderWeele. (2011). Compound treatments and transportability of causal inference. *Epidemiology* **22**(3): 368–377.

Holmberg, S., and A. Thelin. (2013). High dairy fat intake related to less central obesity: a male cohort study with 12 years' follow-up. *Scand J Prim Health Care* **31**(2): 89–94.

Hood, L., and M. Flores. (2012). A personal view on systems medicine and the emergence of proactive P4 medicine: predictive, preventive, personalized and participatory. *N Biotechnol* **29**(6): 613–624.

Huang, J., M. Sherraden, Y. Kim, and M. Clancy. (2014). Effects of child development accounts on early social–emotional development: an experimental test. *JAMA Pediatr* **168**(3): 265–271.

Johns, D. M., R. Bayer, and S. Galea. (2013). Controversial salt report peppered with uncertainty. *Science* **341**(6150): 1063–1064.

Keil, A. P., J. K. Edwards, D. B. Richardson, A. I. Naimi, and S. R. Cole. (2014). The parametric g-formula for time-to-event data: intuition and a worked example. *Epidemiology* **25**(6): 889–897.

Keyes, K., and S. Galea. (2014). Do the results matter beyond the study sample? In *Epidemiology matters: a new introduction to methodological foundations*. K. Keyes and S. Galea, editors. New York: Oxford University Press: 189–197.

Keyes, K. M., and R. Miech. (2013). Commentary on Dawson et al. (2013): drink to your health? Maybe not. *Addiction* **108**(4): 723–724.

Keyes, K. M., G. D. Smith, K. C. Koenen, and S. Galea. (2015). The mathematical limits of genetic prediction for complex chronic disease. *J Epidemiol Community Health* **69**(6): 574–579.

Krieger, N. (1994). Epidemiology and the web of causation: has anyone seen the spider? *Soc Sci Med* **39**(7): 887–903.

Krieger, N. (2011). Does epidemiologic theory exist? In *Epidemiology and the people's health: theory and context*. N. Krieger, editor. New York: Oxford University Press: 3–41.

Krieger, N. (2012). Methods for the scientific study of discrimination and health: an ecosocial approach. *Am J Public Health* **102**(5): 936–944.

Kromhout, D., J. M. Geleijnse, A. Menotti, and D. R. Jacobs, Jr. (2011). The confusion about dietary fatty acids recommendations for CHD prevention. *Br J Nutr* **106**(5): 627–632.

Kuh, D., Y. Ben-Shlomo, J. Lynch, J. Hallqvist, and C. Power. (2003). Life course epidemiology. *J Epidemiol Community Health* **57**(10): 778–783.

Kuhn, T. (1981). *The structure of scientific revolutions*. Chicago: Chicago University Press.

Kuller, L. H. (2013). Point: is there a future for innovative epidemiology? *Am J Epidemiol* **177**(4): 279–280.

Lewis, C. E., K. M. McTigue, L. E. Burke, P. Poirier, R. H. Eckel, B. V. Howard, et al. (2009). Mortality, health outcomes, and body mass index in the overweight range: a science advisory from the American Heart Association. *Circulation* **119**(25): 3263–3271.

Li, K., A. Husing, R. T. Fortner, A. Tjonneland, L. Hansen, L. Dossus, et al. (2015). An epidemiologic risk prediction model for ovarian cancer in Europe: the EPIC study. *Br J Cancer* **112**(7): 1257–1265.

Ludwig, J., and D. A. Phillips. (2008). Long-term effects of Head Start on low-income children. *Ann N Y Acad Sci* **1136**: 257–268.

Maldonado, G., and S. Greenland. (2002). Estimating causal effects. *Int J Epidemiol* **31**(2): 422–429.

Marshall, B. D., and S. Galea. (2015). Formalizing the role of agent-based modeling in causal inference and epidemiology. *Am J Epidemiol* **181**(2): 92–99.

McKeown, R. E. (2009). The epidemiologic transition: changing patterns of mortality and population dynamics. *Am J Lifestyle Med* **3**(1 Suppl): 19S–26S.

McLaughlin, K. A., J. Greif Green, M. J. Gruber, N. A. Sampson, A. M. Zaslavsky, and R. C. Kessler. (2012). Childhood adversities and first onset of psychiatric disorders in a national sample of US adolescents. *Arch Gen Psychiatry* **69**(11): 1151–1160.

Morabia, A. (2014). Tobacco and health: the great controversy. In *Enigmas of health and disease: how epidemiology helps unravel scientific mysteries*. A. Morabia, editor. New York: Columbia University Press: 97–124.

Munoz, I. D., and M. van der Laan. (2012). Population intervention causal effects based on stochastic interventions. *Biometrics* **68**(2): 541–549.

Naimi, A. I., and J. S. Kaufman. (2015). Counterfactual theory in social epidemiology: reconciling analysis and action for the social determinants of health. *Curr Epidemiol Rep* **2**(1): 52–60.

Naimi, A. I., E. E. Moodie, N. Auger, and J. S. Kaufman. (2014). Stochastic mediation contrasts in epidemiologic research: interpregnancy interval and the educational disparity in preterm delivery. *Am J Epidemiol* **180**(4): 436–445.

Nandi, A., M. M. Glymour, and S. V. Subramanian. (2014). Association among socioeconomic status, health behaviors, and all-cause mortality in the United States. *Epidemiology* **25**(2): 170–177.

Park, S. L., I. Cheng, S. A. Pendergrass, A. M. Kucharska-Newton, U. Lim, J. L. Ambite, et al. (2013). Association of the FTO obesity risk variant rs8050136 with percentage of energy intake from fat in multiple racial/ethnic populations: the PAGE study. *Am J Epidemiol* **178**(5): 780–790.

Peng, S., Y. Zhu, F. Xu, X. Ren, X. Li, and M. Lai. (2011). FTO gene polymorphisms and obesity risk: a meta-analysis. *BMC Med* **9**: 71.

Pepe, M. S., H. Janes, G. Longton, W. Leisenring, and P. Newcomb. (2004). Limitations of the odds ratio in gauging the performance of a diagnostic, prognostic, or screening marker. *Am J Epidemiol* **159**(9): 882–890.

Petersen, M. L., S. E. Sinisi, and M. J. van der Laan. (2006). Estimation of direct causal effects. *Epidemiology* **17**(3): 276–284.

Poole, C. (2010). On the origin of risk relativism. *Epidemiology* **21**(1): 3–9.

Popper, K. (1935). *The logic of scientific discovery*. Vienna, Austria: Verlag von Julius Springer.

Ramos, E., S. L. Callier, and C. N. Rotimi. (2012). Why personalized medicine will fail if we stay the course. *Per Med* **9**(8): 839–847.

Robins, J. M., M. A. Hernan, and B. Brumback. (2000). Marginal structural models and causal inference in epidemiology. *Epidemiology* **11**(5): 550–560.

Rockhill, B. (2005). Theorizing about causes at the individual level while estimating effects at the population level: implications for prevention. *Epidemiology* **16**(1): 124–129.

Rose, G. (1985). Sick individuals and sick populations. *Int J Epidemiol* **14**(1): 32–38.

Rose, G. A., Kay-Tee Khaw, and M. G. Marmot. (2008). *Rose's strategy of preventive medicine: the complete original text*. Oxford, Oxford University Press.

Rosenquist, J. N., S. F. Lehrer, A. J. O'Malley, A. M. Zaslavsky, J. W. Smoller, and N. A. Christakis. (2015). Cohort of birth modifies the association between FTO genotype and BMI. *Proc Natl Acad Sci U S A* **112**(2): 354–359.

Rothman, K. J., H. O. Adami, and D. Trichopoulos. (1998). Should the mission of epidemiology include the eradication of poverty? *Lancet* **352**(9130): 810–813.

Sesso, H. D., J. M. Gaziano, D. J. Jenkins, and J. E. Buring. (2007). Strawberry intake, lipids, C-reactive protein, and the risk of cardiovascular disease in women. *J Am Coll Nutr* **26**(4): 303–310.

Shy, C. M. (1997). The failure of academic epidemiology: witness for the prosecution. *Am J Epidemiol* **145**(6): 479–484; discussion 485–477.

Smith, G. D. (2011). Epidemiology, epigenetics and the 'gloomy prospect': embracing randomness in population health research and practice. *Int J Epidemiol* **40**(3): 537–562.

Taubes, G. (1995). Epidemiology faces its limits. *Science* **269**(5221): 164–169.

Terris, M. (1993). The Society for Epidemiologic Research and the future of epidemiology. *J Public Health Policy* **14**(2): 137–148.

VanderWeele, T. J. (2014). A unification of mediation and interaction: a 4-way decomposition. *Epidemiology* **25**(5): 749–761.

VanderWeele, T. J., and M. A. Hernan. (2013). Causal inference under multiple versions of treatment. *J Causal Inference* **1**(1): 1–20.

Wacholder, S. (2005). The impact of a prevention effort on the community. *Epidemiology* **16**(1): 1–3.

Warrington, N. M., L. D. Howe, L. Paternoster, M. Kaakinen, S. Herrala, V. Huikari, et al. (2015). A genome-wide association study of body mass index across early life and childhood. *Int J Epidemiol* **44**(2): 700–712.

Westreich, D. (2014). From exposures to population interventions: pregnancy and response to HIV therapy. *Am J Epidemiol* **179**(7): 797–806.

Xie, Y. (2013). Population heterogeneity and causal inference. *Proc Natl Acad Sci U S A* **110**(16): 6262–6268.

7

Causal Architecture and What Matters Most

QUANTITATIVE EXAMPLES

IN THE PREVIOUS chapter we outlined an approach for identifying the underlying factors that shift population health that focuses on assessing the prevalence of such factors and their co-occurrence with other potential factors of interest. Such an approach uses traditional risk factor identification as a foundation and suggests progressing forward toward a more holistic examination of the complex interactions that predict health both within and across populations, aligning with population health science foundations. In this chapter we provide quantitative examples of the execution of such an approach.

1.0 Understanding the Impact of Prevalent Versus Rare Causes Mathematically

We are often trained to examine the size of the association between a purported exposure and an outcome to decide whether and how much it matters for variation in the outcome. Yet, as we have documented throughout this book, the factors that matter within a population may not be the same as the factors that matter across populations, and our science in population health rests foundationally on this notion. Therefore, any approach

---

Note: Portions of the text in this chapter are adapted from Keyes K. M., and S. Galea. (2015). "What matters most: quantifying an epidemiology of consequence." *Ann Epidemiol* **25**, 305–311.

that analyzes data from a population health science perspective must take into account the factors that differ within and across populations. To do so, the fundamental principle that should guide our work is that the determination of the size of an association is dependent on the prevalence of the co-occurring causes that interact to produce health indicators in populations.

To illustrate these concepts, we created a series of examples that shows, through simple mathematical manipulation, several critical principles that underlie how we should think about assessing causation in population health science.

1.1   Example 1: The Same Set of Causes Can Produce Different Causal Effects Across Populations

We construct a hypothetical disease that has three causes: E, W, and Z. E and W interact to produce disease (the only individuals who develop disease through E are those who also have W), and Z is a set of causes that does not include E or W. Suppose we are interested in assessing whether E is associated with disease.

We examine the effect of E on disease in two populations. In Table 7.1, we show the number of individuals in the population who have E, W, and Z, and whether they have the disease (i.e., those with both E and W, and those with Z). In both populations, there is an equal proportion of people who have Z; thus, there is a comparable percentage of exposed and unexposed individuals who get the disease through causes that do not involve exposure to E. The populations also have the same prevalence of E; the only difference between the two populations is the prevalence of exposure to W. Prevalence is 30% in population 1 and 60% in population 2. In population 1, those with E have 1.5 times the risk of disease, and exposure to E is associated with 10 additional cases per 100 exposed. This is a causal estimate. In population 2, exposure to disease is associated with three times the risk of disease and E is associated with 40 additional cases per 100 exposed. This, too, is a causal estimate. In sum, E is associated with many more cases of disease per 100 people in population 2 compared with population 1.

Thus, we have two different populations with two different causal effects, and the reason they differ is the prevalence of W. We will have a limited understanding of how many cases of disease will be prevented if we block E unless we know the prevalence of W. Furthermore, co-occurring cause prevalence determines the magnitude of a causal effect of an exposure; the

Table 7.1 Two Populations with the Same Prevalence of Exposure But Different Causal Effects of Exposure on Disease

	Population 1					Population 2		
	D+	D–	N			D+	D–	N
E+	30	70	100		E+	60	40	100
E–	20	80	100		E–	20	80	100
N	50	150	200		N	80	120	200

				D?	N					D?	N
E	W	Z		1	20	E	W	Z		1	20
E	W–	Z		1	0	E	W–	Z		1	0
E	W	Z–		1	10	E	W	Z–		1	40
E	W–	Z–		0	70	E	W–	Z–		0	40
E–	W–	Z–		0	50	E–	W–	Z–		0	20
E–	W	Z–		0	30	E–	W	Z–		0	60
E–	W–	Z		1	20	E–	W–	Z		1	20
E–	W	Z		1	0	E–	W	Z		1	0
					200						200
			RR	1.50					RR	3.00	
			RD	0.10					RD	0.40	

RD, relative difference; RR, relative risk.

exposure has the same prevalence in the two populations, and yet different magnitudes of effect because of the changing prevalence of W.

1.2 Example 2: A Different Set of Causes Can Produce the Same Causal Effect Across Populations

In contrast to example 1, we may also encounter situations in which the causal effect is the same in two different populations but the distribution of co-occurring causes differs. In Table 7.2, we again have two different populations, and different distributions of E, W, and Z co-occurrence across these populations (e.g., there are 20 individuals in population 1 exposed to E and Z but not W, whereas there are 30 individuals of this type in population 2). These distributions generate the same numbers in our two-by-two table, and thus the same risk ratio and risk difference. E is associated with a 1.5 increase

102 POPULATION HEALTH SCIENCE

Table 7.2 Two Populations with the Same Causal Effect of Exposure on Disease But Different Distributions of Component Causes

	Population 1					Population 2			
	D+	D−	N			D+	D−	N	
E+	60	20	80		E+	60	20	80	
E−	40	40	80		E−	40	40	80	
N	100	60	160		N	100	60	160	

			D?	N				D?	N
E	W	Z	1	20	E	W	Z	1	10
E	W−	Z	1	20	E	W−	Z	1	30
E	W	Z−	1	20	E	W	Z−	1	20
E	W−	Z−	0	20	E	W−	Z−	0	20
E−	W−	Z−	0	20	E−	W−	Z−	0	20
E−	W	Z−	0	20	E−	W	Z−	0	20
E−	W−	Z	1	20	E−	W−	Z	1	30
E−	W	Z	1	20	E−	W	Z	1	10
				160					160
			RR	1.50				RR	1.50
			RD	0.25				RD	0.25

RD, relative difference; RR, relative risk.

in risk, and an additional 25 cases per 100 exposed. However, the underlying causal structures in the two populations that result in these measures of association are different. In population 1 compared with population 2, there are more cases that have all three exposures: E, W, and Z. Thus, removal of E would not influence disease in these people. Again, the difference between the two populations is the prevalence of W. Without knowing the prevalence of W, we cannot fully determine the magnitude of the impact of E, because it varies depending on whether or not W is present.

1.3 Example 3: Understanding Differing Causal Effects Across Populations Using the Example of Cognitive Ability

To draw from an example in the literature, suppose we are interested in whether a set of genes influences cognitive ability (Rutter 2007, Swanson et al. 2015). At least some proportion of the variability in cognitive ability in populations is a result of the genetic factors passed down from parents to offspring (Plomin and Spinath 2004, Deary et al. 2006). However, a supporting and nurturing early-childhood rearing environment is also important, and some evidence indicates such environments potentiate the effects of what we might term the "genetic endowment" of the child (Neisser et al. 1996, Nisbett et al. 2012). Thus, both the genetic material we receive from our biological parents and a supportive environment for nurturing our innate ability matter for the development of cognitive ability.

Suppose we have two populations: one in which exposure to high-quality education is almost ubiquitous (99%) and one in which only the wealthiest 20% of children are exposed to high-quality education. We dichotomize cognitive ability, considering those with high scores on a standardized test to have demonstrated high cognitive ability. We know that cognitive ability exists on a continuous dimension, reflecting that population health manifests as a continuum (foundational principle 1), but here we dichotomize cognitive ability for pedagogical purposes to create a simple example. The central themes illustrated here hold whether the health outcome is dichotomous or observed continuously in populations.

In both populations, approximately 15% of children are born with a genetic endowment that provides the potential to have high cognitive ability. In our example, we assume that genetic endowment is more likely to lead to cognitive ability in the context of high-quality education. However, 5% of children will have high cognitive ability regardless of whether they have a genetic endowment or a supportive learning environment; in other words, among those with no high-quality education, some students will beat the odds and develop cognitive ability. Furthermore, among those with high-quality education, some students will fail to thrive regardless of their genetic endowment.

Results of such an example are shown in Table 7.3. Although genetic endowment is associated with higher cognitive ability in both populations, the contribution of genetic endowment to cognitive ability in the population with a near-ubiquitous nurturing educational environment is dramatically higher than the contribution of genetic endowment to cognitive ability in the population with lower exposure to a nurturing educational environment. Those with high genetic endowment are almost four times more likely to have high cognitive ability than those in the ubiquitous nurturing learning environment; in contrast, when the prevalence of nurturing learning environment exposure is low, those with the genetic endowment are about 1.4 times more likely to have high cognitive ability.

Note again, the prevalence of genetic endowment and the structure of how cognitive ability is caused is the same in the two populations; the only

Table 7.3 The Association Between Genetic Factors and Cognitive Ability in Two Populations*

99% of Children in Nurturing Educational Environment				RR	3.99
	CA+	CA−	Total	RD	0.15
GE+	303	1214	1517	RD	0.75
GE−	425	8060	8485		
Total	728	9274	10,002		
20% of Children in Nurturing Educational Environment				RR	1.43
	CA+	RD	Total	RD	0.0210
GE+	110	RD	1517	PARP	0.30
GE−	430	8055	8485		
Total	540	9462	10,002		

* In population 1, 99% of children are exposed to a nurturing educational environment. In population 2, 20% of children are exposed to a nurturing educational environment. RD, risk difference; RR, risk ratio.

thing that changed was the environment. This suggests that when all children are in a nurturing environment, genetic endowments to high cognitive ability become the principal reason that separates high from low cognitive achievers. In contrast, when a minority of children are exposed to a nurturing environment, it is much more difficult to see contributions to cognitive ability from genetic endowment, and whether a child does have such an endowment matters much less in explaining population health.

In fact, the empirical literature on differences in the heritability of cognitive ability across learning environments suggests the same results we simulated here. Using twin data, Turkheimer et al. (2003) demonstrated the proportion of variance in intelligence explained by genetics was highest among children in the highest socioeconomic strata. As the socioeconomic stratum declines, the contribution of additive genetic effects decreases whereas the contribution of a shared environment increases. Although follow-up studies have shown inconsistencies in these findings across development and context (Rutter 2007), it is clear that the contribution of specific causes to variation in cognitive ability differ systematically across contexts in which the co-occurring causes also vary. Thus, understanding cognitive ability requires an approach that seeks to understand the way in which these causes work together, rather than estimating the specific causal effect of any one cause.

2.0 Co-occurrence of Causes and Their Impact on Population Health Science Assessment

These examples illustrate that understanding nature through isolating the effects of single causes on health indicators is often limited by the consistency of the prevalence of co-occurring causes across populations in which we want to intervene. This notion is well documented in epidemiological and causal inference literature, often grouped under the rubric of factors that affect "transportability" (Cole and Stuart 2010, Hernan and VanderWeele 2011, Pearl and Bareinboim 2011), or generalizability. Although assessing the effects of single factors on health (e.g. "risk factors") has been the bedrock of science and in public health, and has led to a deep understanding of many important causes, we cannot escape the fact that studies of humans in their environments inevitably require frameworks that allow for articulating and modeling the dynamic ways in which individuals interact with each other and their exposures differently depending on time, place, and person. This is not, to be sure, a criticism of the methods we use to specify precise causal effects. Such methods force us to be rigorous in our thinking and in our questioning. Rather, we suggest that a reframing of the questions and, subsequently, the methods that illuminate the drivers of population health, is required.

In sum, the examples we show in this chapter illustrate our sixth foundational principle of population health science (Box 7.1).

For some exposure–outcome relations, the prevalence of interacting factors may be relatively constant across populations. For example, the association between smoking and lung cancer is relatively consistent (or, at least, always very strong [Lee et al. 2012]), indicating the factors that interact with smoking to produce lung cancer have a relatively homogenous prevalence across many populations. Yet, even with smoking and lung cancer there have been numerous factors that have been identified that interact with smoking and vary the magnitude of the association (Saracci 1987). If these factors vary in prevalence across

---

BOX 7.1

Sixth Foundational Principle of Population Health Science

The magnitude of an effect of exposure on disease is dependent on the prevalence of factors that interact with that exposure.

populations, we would expect the magnitude of association between smoking and lung cancer to vary. Thus, the magnitudes of our associations are bound in time and place, and the magnitudes of our measures of association are bounded by the dynamics of the environments in which they were estimated (Schwartz et al. 2011). The magnitude of a causal effect now may no longer apply in the future if the population is dynamic enough.

3.0 From Simulation to the Community: Shifting Exposure Prevalence Across Geographic Space and Time

One could potentially write off our previous examples as convenient mathematical exercises, but there is substantial empirical literature to indicate such variations in the magnitudes of our effect estimates occur frequently. These variations are sometimes explained by random chance (Ioannidis 2005, Smith 2011), faulty study design, or other methodological bias, and such explanations citing methodological bias expose our preference for effects that are universal, because they offer perhaps simpler or easy-to-explain associations and potential public health interventions.

The most obvious areas in public health in which we see variation in the magnitudes of effect of exposures on disease across contexts include infectious diseases. For example, consider the basic and net reproductive rate, central measures of the average number of additional cases per infected person, in which the former is estimated among a completely susceptible population whereas the latter can vary according to vaccination and other sources of immunity. Although the basic reproductive rate provides some information about the underlying pathogenesis and virulence of infection, the net reproductive rate is expected to vary widely across geographic contexts, subpopulations, and time as immunity levels change within and across populations. Thus, built into the assessment of infectious disease transmission and incidence is an explicit understanding of the way in which context and distributions of risk and protective factors alter our estimates of disease pathogenesis.

As another example, consider firearm violence in the United States. Death by gun violence is among one of the most central threats currently facing public health in the United States. One response to the threat has been to restrict the purchase and carrying of firearms by individuals with mental illness. In fact, firearm-disqualifying mental health adjudications increased from 7% in 2007 to 28% in 2013 (Swanson et al. 2015). When we step back from the United States and compare across countries, however, we see that, in comparison, Canada has a similar prevalence of psychiatric disorders compared with the United States (Bland et al. 1988, Offord et al. 1996, Kessler et al. 2005), but a much lower overall rate of gun violence and a much smaller proportion of homicides and suicides committed with guns (Navaneelan 2009). In fact, empirical evidence from the United States indicates there is only a marginal association between mental illness and increased risk of violence (Glied and Frank 2014, Swanson et al. 2015), suggesting the dynamics that underlie the epidemic of firearm injury in the United States require little focus on mental illness. Differences in firearm availability and gun culture may underlie the differences in firearm injury across these two geographic contexts (Miller et al. 2002), and a focus on factors such as mental illness may misplace resources. Understanding the causal architecture of firearm violence and the factors that vary across geographic contexts (e.g., firearm availability, [Hepburn & Hemenway 2004]) and those that do not (e.g., mental illness prevalence) provides a framework that draws attention to the areas in which the greatest public health impact could be found.

We can draw on many more examples from the literature to illustrate this foundational point: the variation in the magnitudes of our associations across time and place are a critical part of the epidemiology of our outcomes and, by drawing on this variation, we may be able to acquire a stronger foothold into how we can shift population health more dramatically.

Furthermore, understanding the shifting magnitudes of association across populations as a foothold into causal architecture is not the only way to increase our capacity for a population health science of consequence. A deeper engagement with the mechanisms through which exposures (prevalent or rare) exert an impact can provide insight into the more generalizable processes through which health is distributed across populations (Shadish et al. 2002, Broadbent 2013). The need to "look inside the black box" to formulate a science that explicates general mechanisms beyond context-specific mechanisms underscores central philosophical tensions about the role of epidemiology as a science. However, more instrumentally, methods and applications of mediation within the epidemiological context are developing rapidly, providing us with an opportunity to shed light on mechanisms that can inform our science (De Stavola et al. 2015, Nandi et al. 2014, VanderWeele 2014, Albert and Wang 2015). We suggest that methods and applications of context-specific approaches that endeavor to outline the ways in which, and the reasons why, associations differ across context should be a useful adjunct to these developing methodologies.

4.0 References

Albert, J. M., and W. Wang. (2015). Sensitivity analyses for parametric causal mediation effect estimation. *Biostatistics* **16**(2): 339–351.

Bland, R. C., S. C. Newman, and H. Orn. (1988). Period prevalence of psychiatric disorders in Edmonton. *Acta Psychiatr Scand Suppl* **338**: 33–42.

Broadbent, A. (2013). *Philosophy of epidemiology.* London: Palgrave Macmillan.

Cole, S. R., and E. A. Stuart. (2010). Generalizing evidence from randomized clinical trials to target populations: the ACTG 320 trial. *Am J Epidemiol* **172**(1): 107–115.

Deary, I. J., F. M. Spinath, and T. C. Bates. (2006). Genetics of intelligence. *Eur J Hum Genet* **14**(6): 690–700.

De Stavola, B. L., R. M. Daniel, G. B. Ploubidis, and N. Micali. (2015). Mediation analysis with intermediate confounding: structural equation modeling viewed through the causal inference lens. *Am J Epidemiol* **181**(1): 64–80.

Glied, S., and R. G. Frank. (2014). Mental illness and violence: lessons from the evidence. *Am J Public Health* **104**(2): e5–e6.

Hepburn, L. M., and D. Hemenway (2004). Firearm availability and homicide: A review of the literature. *Aggression and Violent Behavior* **9**(4): 417–440.

Hernan, M. A., and T. J. VanderWeele. (2011). Compound treatments and transportability of causal inference. *Epidemiology* **22**(3): 368–377.

Ioannidis, J. P. A. (2005). Why most published research findings are false. *PLoS Med* **2**(8): e124.

Kessler, R. C., P. Berglund, O. Demler, R. Jin, K. R. Merikangas, and E. E. Walters. (2005). Lifetime prevalence and age-of-onset distributions of DSM-IV disorders in the National Comorbidity Survey Replication. *Arch Gen Psychiatry* **62**(6): 593–602.

Lee, P. N., B. A. Forey, and K. J. Coombs. (2012). Systematic review with meta-analysis of the epidemiological evidence in the 1900s relating smoking to lung cancer. *BMC Cancer* **12**: 385.

Miller, M., D. Azrael, and D. Hemenway. (2002). Firearm availability and unintentional firearm deaths, suicide, and homicide among 5–14 year olds. *J Trauma* **52**(2): 267–274; discussion 274–265.

Nandi, A., M. M. Glymour, and S. V. Subramanian. (2014). Association among socioeconomic status, health behaviors, and all-cause mortality in the United States. *Epidemiology* **25**(2): 170–177.

Navaneelan, T. (2009). *Suicide rates: an overview.* Available: http://www.statcan.gc.ca/pub/82-624-x/2012001/article/11696-eng.htm.

Neisser, U., G. Boodoo, T. Bouchard, A. W. Boykin, N. Brody, S. J. Ceci, et al. (1996). Intelligence: knowns and unknowns. *Am Psychol* **51**(2): 77–101.

Nisbett, R. E., J. Aronson, C. Blair, W. Dickens, J. Flynn, D. F. Halpern, et al. (2012). Intelligence: new findings and theoretical developments. *Am Psychol* **67**(2): 130–159.

Offord, D. R., M. H. Boyle, D. Campbell, P. Goering, E. Lin, M. Wong, et al. (1996). One-year prevalence of psychiatric disorder in Ontarians 15 to 64 years of age. *Can J Psychiatry* **41**(9): 559–563.

Pearl, J., and E. Bareinboim. (2011). Transportability of causal and statistical relations: a formal approach. In *Proceedings of the 25th AAAI Conference on Artificial Intelligence*. Menlo Park, CA: AAAI Press: 247–254.

Plomin, R., and F. M. Spinath. (2004). Intelligence: genetics, genes, and genomics. *J Pers Soc Psychol* 86(1): 112–129.

Rutter, M. (2007). Gene–environment interdependence. *Dev Sci* 10(1): 12–18.

Saracci, R. (1987). The interactions of tobacco smoking and other agents in cancer etiology. *Epidemiol Rev* 9: 175–193.

Schwartz, S., N. Gatto, and U. Campbell (2011). What would have been is not what would be: counterfactuals of the past and potential outcomes of the future. In *Causality and psychopathology*. P. Shrout, K. Keyes, and K. Ornstein, editors. New York: Oxford University Press: 25–46.

Shadish, W. R., T. D. Cook, and D. T. Campbel. (2002). Construct validity and external validity. In *Experimental and quasi-experimental designs for generalized causal inferences* (2nd edition). W. R. Shadish, T. D. Cook, and D. T. Campbel, editors. Boston, MA: Houghton Mifflin: 64–102.

Smith, G. D. (2011). Epidemiology, epigenetics and the 'gloomy prospect': embracing randomness in population health research and practice. *Int J Epidemiol* 40(3): 537–562.

Swanson, J. W., E. E. McGinty, S. Fazel, and V. M. Mays. (2015). Mental illness and reduction of gun violence and suicide: bringing epidemiologic research to policy. *Ann Epidemiol* 25(5): 366–376.

Turkheimer, E., A. Haley, M. Waldron, B. D'Onofrio, and I. I. Gottesman. (2003). Socioeconomic status modifies heritability of IQ in young children. *Psychol Sci* 14(6): 623–628.

VanderWeele, T. J. (2014). A unification of mediation and interaction: a 4-way decomposition. *Epidemiology* 25(5): 749–761.

8

Valuing Population Health Interventions

MEASURING RETURN ON INVESTMENT

IN THIS CHAPTER we focus on an approach that is at the core of population health science: an understanding of health return on investment (ROI) and a recognition that the maximizing of population health is likelier to find foothold if it stands on a robust demonstration of approaches that maximize such return. We note that population health science is concerned explicitly with the health ROI rather than the monetary ROI from intervention. Although monetary ROI and cost-effectiveness are important to consider, we focus here on health returns, given the centrality of improving population health to our particular science.

This chapter both builds on our quest for a causal architecture that allows us to engage in consequential science and also builds on our discussion about macrosocial determinants in Chapter 5. As we recognize the centrality of large-scale social, cultural, political, and economic ubiquitous factors in shaping population health, it is inevitable that we must grapple with questions about the ROI that might accompany efforts to change these large-scale factors.

The concept of ROI is used in a broad array of disciplines—most notably, the financial world. Investors in a new business, for example, expect that for each dollar they provide to the developers, they will reap more than the dollar in a certain amount of time. The ROI, then, is the number of dollars reaped for each dollar provided initially. We can conceptualize ROI in general as follows:

$$\mathrm{ROI} = \frac{\mathrm{Current\ Value - Cost\ of\ Investment}}{\mathrm{Cost\ of\ Investment}}$$

For example, if Susan purchases $100 of shares in Big Business Inc., and 1 year later she sells the shares for $150, then her ROI over 1 year is ($150 − $100)/100 = 0.5 or 50%. The financial concept of ROI allows us to quantitatively assess the current value of an asset versus the initial cost. Suppose for example, that Juan sells shares in Toy Makers Inc. for $5000 after 1 year and brags to Susan that he made more money than her. If his initial cost for the shares was $4000, then his ROI is ($5000 − 4000)/4000 = 0.25, or 25%. Thus, although Juan has more money than Susan at the end of 1 year, he made a lower return on his investment than Susan.

These concepts are basic principles of investing and finance, but can be applied equally to the study of population health as we consider whether and where to place public and private resources to improve health. In this chapter we outline basic principles of ROI for population health interventions. We note that the analytic field of ROI and related concepts such as cost-effectiveness analyses have grown rapidly and matured in quantitative sophistication, and this chapter does not endeavor to be a full and detailed guide to applying complex ROI modeling. Instead, we provide here an overview of basic theoretical concepts and their application to provide you with the basic tools of how to think about ROI as a function of population health science. As noted earlier, this chapter does not consider monetary ROIs or cost effectiveness. Again, we focus the discussion in this chapter on how to consider improving population health, as this is a central concept in public health policy and evaluation. We would endeavor to have such improvements be cost-effective and efficacious, but our focus in population health science is in bringing about health change. We conclude the chapter by showing how prevention approaches maximize ROI for population health, suggesting the importance of a focus on prevention as the remit of population health inquiry and practice.

1.0 Return on Investment for Health: An Overview

Unlike the financial investor who aims to build wealth, in return on health investment we strive to build health. The basic issue is how much health is gained from each dollar spent on a particular course of action (or inaction). The answer to this issue depends on a number of parameters, including whose dollars are being invested, the cost of the initial investment, where and when the money is spent during the life course, how long we anticipate the return to accrue, the opportunity cost of one particular course of action

Valuing Population Health Interventions: Measuring Return on Investment 113

versus another, and what we mean by "health." Each of these parameters must be considered as we endeavor to evaluate where health investments should be placed.

1.1 Measuring End Points in Returns on Health Investments

When we move from a financial model to a health model, the basic parameters of the ROI formula become more complicated. In the financial model, the ultimate goal is to build wealth for investors. They take a risk by investing money and, hopefully, reap a monetary reward for that risk. What is the reward in population health? Is it increasing the number of years lived? Is it reducing the number of cases of a certain illness? Or, is it decreasing a problematic health behavior (e.g., smoking)? Each of these potential end points has its own set of complexities in terms of effect estimation.

Furthermore, the ROI must take into consideration who or what we conceptualize to be the investor, or the stakeholder of interest. In classic financial investment, payers puts their money at risk and then (hopefully) reap the rewards for that risk. In population health, the actual cost of the investment may come from multiple and diverse sources, including ministries or departments of health, employers, universities, private companies, or community-based organizations. The ROI can then be described in terms of actual health benefits, costs benefits, or a number of other metrics. For example, suppose we want to know the ROI for providing subsidized gym memberships through employers. One metric might be how many fewer heart attacks there are in the population during a certain time period, but another might be how many fewer sick days there are among employees of a certain business. In addition to the occurrence or incidence of specific health events during a circumscribed time period (see "The Value of Prevention: The Impact of Interventions over Time" later in this chapter), or all-cause and cause-specific mortality, commonly used metrics for measuring ROI for a particular population health initiative include the disability-adjusted life year (DALY) and the quality-adjusted life year (QALY).

1.2 Disability-Adjusted Life Years

When we seek to improve the population's health through intervention, one way we can estimate the potential (or realized) return for population health is through the number of DALYs gained through a particular intervention. The disability adjusted life years associated with the occurrence of sickness, disease, symptoms, or syndromes refers simultaneously to two components: the years of life lost (YLL) and the years lost as a result of disability (YLD). YLL can be conceptualized as a measure of the number of additional years an individual would have survived without the presence or level of the particular health indicator. YLD can be conceptualized as the years of productive life lost as a result of reduced functioning because of the particular health indicator. For example, if an individual survives but cannot participate in normal functions of daily life because of illness, this lack of productivity would be counted as YLD. We should note that "normal" functions depend on a host of values at the societal level and the means of accommodations in a society for individuals with a range of abilities. If individuals die as a result of the illness, obviously they can no longer be productive in daily life, and those years lost are counted as YLL. The basic equation for YLL is

$$YLL = N \times L,$$

where N is the number of deaths attributable to the health indicator of interest in a specific population in a given year and L is the difference between the average life expectancy in the overall population and the average age of death among those who died of the disease under study. For example, in a population of 100,000 individuals, if 500 deaths are attributable to HIV/acquired immune deficiency syndrome (AIDS) and those 500 people had an average age of death of 60 years compared with the population average life expectancy of 80 years, the YLL is (80 − 60) × 500. Thus, there are 10,000 years of life lost from HIV/AIDS in this population. When we assess YLD, the parameters change to

$$YLD = I \times L \times DW,$$

where I is the number of incident (i.e., new) cases involving the health indicator, L is the average duration of the disease or other health indicator, and DW is a disability weight. A disability weight is an empirically determined measure of the severity of a health indicator on a scale of zero to one, with zero being no effect on health and one being death. Thus, a disease that does not cause immediate death but reduces ability to function in daily life receives a disability weight greater than zero and less than one. The YLD would then increase in proportion to the duration of the disease and the number of incident cases.

Continuing with our previous example, assuming that, in a given population, there are 100 incident cases of HIV/AIDS in a year, an average duration of illness of 10 years, and a disability weight of about 0.14, the YLD is 140. Thus, there are 140 years lost from disability associated with HIV/AIDS in this population.

Using the YLD and the YLL, we then estimate the DALYs associated with a particular health indicator as

$$DALYs = YLD + YLL.$$

That is, the sum of YLL and YLD forms the DALYs resulting from a health indicator of interest. In our example, the DALYs would be 10,000 + 140, or 10,140 DALYs lost as a result of HIV/AIDS.

When considering a potential intervention and the effects on DALYs, we would compare the population burden of the health indicator (through the DALYs) with the intervention, and the population burden of the health indicator without the intervention. Note the relation between an intervention and DALYs saved may be linear, latent, or nonlinear, or take many functional forms. We provide an example of this later.

For example, DALYs have been used to evaluate the return on health investment of large-scale programs such as antiretroviral treatment (ART) programs for individuals living with HIV/AIDS worldwide. A study funded by the Global Fund to Fight AIDS, Tuberculosis, and Malaria estimated that investment in ART would save about 18.5 million life years between 2011 and 2020, in addition to considerable monetary savings (in the form of increased labor productivity and decreased costs associated with orphan care, opportunistic infection treatment, and end-of-life care) for the nearly 3.5 million individuals in low- and middle-income countries receiving ART treatment co-financed by the Global Fund (Resch et al. 2011).

As another example, harm reduction approaches to IV drug use have been a matter of considerable controversy, yet available data indicate there are substantial health benefits to programs such as clean needle exchanges in reducing infectious disease transmission. In Australia, the government investment in needle and syringe programs from 2000 to 2009 resulted in an estimated gain of approximately 140,000 DALYs and prevented the occurrence of 32,050 new HIV cases and 96,667 new hepatitis C cases (as well as significant financial savings, especially when compared with more traditional interventions such as inpatient treatment programs and vaccinations) (Wilson et al. 2009).

It is important to note that the DALY as a measure of disease burden in populations has been criticized when there is a lack of empirical information on which to base parameter estimates. An accurate measure of DALYs requires knowledge of the incidence and duration of illness, the average age of death among those with the health indicator, and the average overall life expectancy of the population. Each of these parameters can be difficult to estimate accurately without large-scale data collection projects. Even when these parameters are known, estimating the disability weight can be difficult, and empirical data on which to base the weight can be hard to identify. Furthermore, accurate DALYs require causal attribution; that is, we need to specify how many deaths and how much disability are attributable directly to the health indicator. Diseases and other illnesses often co-occur, and it is difficult to attribute death and disability correctly to a specific cause. For example, if an obese individual dies after a myocardial infarction, is the death attributable to obesity or myocardial infarction? Because of the co-occurrence of many diseases and other health indicators of interest, DALYs are often overestimated for any particular disease or health indicator.

1.3 Quality-Adjusted Life Years

The QALY is an alterative way of estimating the potential efficacy of an intervention by taking into consideration not only the reduced time an individual lives or is productive because of an illness or health indicator, but also the quality of the years that are survived in terms of functional capacity, pain, and perception of health. That is, even if an individual lives an additional 5 years because of an intervention, the quality of those years may be diminished if the individual is in serious pain or is unable to perform valued functions in daily life. Thus, the QALY provides a quantitative estimate of the number of additional life years that are somewhat defined amorphously as "quality" years. Developed conceptually during the 1970s (Fanshel and Bush 1970, Torrance 1970, Torrance et al. 1972, Zeckhauser and Shepard 1976), the measure is used in various ways with various metrics for quality that still remain in development.

Defining quality of life is a field in and of itself, and has as much to do with individual perceptions, social norms, and environment as it does with the actual conditions under consideration. It is intuitive that losing the ability to walk as a result of contracting the polio virus at a young age, for example, would have a significant impact on quality of life. However, there have been vast improvements in access for individuals with different capacities for mobility in many countries during the past several decades, thus the impact of losing the ability to walk on quality of life is vastly different in 2015 than it was in 1950. Consider, too, the consumer movements for conditions such as deafness. Although once considered a significant disability, populations within and outside the deaf community consider deafness to be an identity, and advocate for improvements to the environment to allow deaf individuals to thrive rather than to require deaf people to adapt to an environment designed for hearing populations.

QALYs are estimated by multiplying a year of life by a weighting factor that indicates how much utility, functionality, or impairment occurs during the year:

$$QALY = 1 \times w,$$

where 1 is a year time period and w is a weight that refers to the utility of that year in terms of quality of life. In general, we conceptualize this utility on a line from one to zero, where one is perfect health and zero is death.

The determination of the magnitude of this weighting factor is derived through a number of different metrics, including scales that describe functional impairments. One commonly used metric is a time tradeoff, whereby individuals are asked whether they would prefer to remain in various states of health (average, poor, bedridden, unconscious, and so on) for a period of time versus remaining in perfect health but having a shorter life expectancy. Other common metrics are used to describe various medical procedures that may either cure or kill versus remaining in a specific state of health. As an example, if I bumped into a table and had a bruise on my leg, I would choose to remain in that state of health for a week rather than elect for a medical intervention that may cure the bruise but might kill me. If I had late-stage cancer, however, I might chose a risky medical intervention knowing that the chance of survival is less than perfect. It is also important to note that QALYs can be negative; some conditions are rated by patients on average as being less preferable than death (e.g., conditions in which the individual is unresponsive, confined to a bed, or unable to communicate).

The QALY as a measure of ROI has faced criticism in the literature, given that there is substantial variation at the population level in terms of what is quality life. That is, if we asked individuals to rate where on the number line between one (perfect health) and zero (death) they would place a condition that involved moderate depression with some chronic pain, one person might rate that health state as 0.25 whereas someone else might rate it as 0.5. Overall, there is no empirical constant for the quality of a life year given certain symptoms and challenges because "quality" of life is a subjective concept. Even the concept of "perfect health" likely differs from person to person. Thus, given a large enough sample size in which quality ratings are assessed, we obtain the population average with substantial error for the assessment of a QALY. Furthermore, most QALY estimates include a discounting rate (described later in the chapter) that can also be difficult to parameterize empirically (for a more detailed discussion of formulas to parameterize QALY, there are several comprehensive explanations in the literature [Prieto and Sacristan 2003, Sassi 2006]).

2.0 The Value of Prevention: The Impact of Interventions over Time

Prevention of disease and the promotion of health are at the heart of population health science. The reasons for this start with our values. Broadly speaking, we would rather not develop disease at all than develop disease and need to be treated for it. Ask yourself: Would you rather live in a world where very few people develop schizophrenia or live in a world with effective treatments for schizophrenia? Clearly, prevention is more optimal than effective treatment, although when complete prevention is currently impossible, effective treatment is critical. Therefore, prevention represents an important corollary focus for population health science and represents a core stratagem of population health. However, prevention is often difficult, strategies for complex chronic diseases are underdeveloped, and prevention efforts face the "prevention paradox" discussed in Chapter 3: what is good for the population may not be good for the individual, because we do not know which individuals would have developed the disease in the absence of the preventive intervention.

The approaches central to valuing population health discussed here, and the centrality of preventive approaches therein, are elevated by several concepts that are fundamental to consider simultaneously: lag time, compounding "interest," and discounting rates. We discuss each in turn next.

We would like to see benefits accrue from our action on a relatively proximal timescale. However, for some of the biggest "wins" in population health, particularly for preventive interventions, immediacy is not always possible or even optimal. Investment in early-childhood education (Schweinhart 1993, Karoly and Levaux 1998), child and adolescent campaigns to prevent smoking onset and other drug use (Bruvold 1993, Tobler et al. 2000), or in green space and land use (Lee and Maheswaran 2011), for example, are all efforts to prevent disease that may have long-ranging effects throughout the life course of individuals exposed to such interventions in ways that cannot be captured in a 1-year, 5-year, or even a 10-year follow-up period. The lag time creates ambiguities and complications for assessing the effects of such interventions on health: other interventions and exposures may change across the same period, investment in the study of long-ranging effects is expensive and time-consuming, and exposures with long lag periods may have diffuse and difficult-to-measure consequences, both positive and negative. Yet, these methodological and logistical challenges should not preclude the consideration of preventive interventions with long lag times; they only make our job as population health scientists that much more challenging. For example, Heckman and others (Heckman 2000, Heckman 2006, Heckman 2007, Cunha et al. 2010) have argued that early-childhood intervention on cognitive ability may have benefits that accrue across the life span, such that assessment of success or failure of such interventions during early childhood is insufficient to capture the total effects. Thus, for any preventive or population health intervention, a full articulation of short-, middle-, and long-term anticipated consequences and benefits are critical to evaluation efforts.

Potential long-term outcomes of preventive population health interventions are complicated to conceptualize for a number of critical reasons that are fundamental to understanding potential returns on such investments. The distribution of long-ranging consequences across time may not be constant. A clear example of this is in the concept of compound interest, familiar in the financial literature and applicable conceptually to population health science. Consider an investment of $100 that returns 10% each year. After 1 year, we would have $110. That $110 then becomes reinvested, and after 2 years becomes $121. After 3 years, we have $133.10. Thus, we make interest on the interest that has already accrued after 1 year. The same concept can be applied conceptually to health. If we analyze only the benefit of a health intervention after a short time, we may not realize the long-ranging and compounded potential health benefits throughout an extended time frame. For example, an intervention to promote early-childhood nutrition may have a positive impact on rates of childhood obesity in the short term; however, preventing childhood obesity could have long-ranging effects on adolescent and adult obesity above and beyond what we would anticipate if we were to conduct the same intervention at a later time in the life course. This concept is akin to concepts of critical periods and accumulation of risk models we discussed in Chapter 4. That is, intervention at a critical time point in development may interact with other exposures and developmental processes that portend greater health benefits than intervention at a later time point in an individual's development.

Furthermore, population heath interventions themselves, more broadly—and preventive interventions, specifically—may not have a linear effect on health returns. For example, a concept often invoked in economics discussions is that of synergy or dynamic complementarities between early interventions and later interventions, or between multiple simultaneous interventions. For those in the quantitative health sciences, this is akin to the concept of interaction, or the life course concept of accumulation of risk that we discussed in Chapter 4. That is, for some interventions, there may be later interventions that are needed to augment the effects of early interventions. Those later interventions themselves, without the early interventions, may have less or no impact on population health. Thus, the synergy or interaction between the early and later interventions together has an impact on improving population health. An intuitive example of this is booster shots for vaccination. The benefits of early vaccination to prevent disease are compounded by "boosters" at later ages. The boosters themselves have little impact without the early vaccinations. Moving beyond the vaccination example, Heckman (2008) described such a process for the effects of early-childhood education; one-time investments are not enough for maximum impact. If early investments are followed up with later (less expensive) investments, the investments compound and become synergistic. Although in life course processes we often consider accumulation of risk to be the way in which risks that occur at various points in the life course can together bring about an adverse health outcome at a later time point, in this context we would consider interventions that occur at various points in the life course to work together to bring out the maximum benefit or return on population health.

ROI models can also follow other life course models, such as those discussed in Chapter 4. For example, self-productivity refers to an intervention to increase capacity at time t, which in turn leads to a greater ability to increase capacity at time $t + 1$. This is similar to the chains of risk model discussed in Chapter 4. That is, an intervention at a particular time point sets forth a cascade of activity in which exposures (or additional interventions) that occur later in the life course are the result of that initial exposure itself. Taken together, the concepts described in this section make clear our suggestion that prevention of disease has a greater ROI than curing disease after it has started, through long-range and latent effects, complementarities, and compounded returns.

Together, these diffusive effects form the foundation that makes preventive interventions among the more fruitful paths for improving population

Valuing Population Health Interventions: Measuring Return on Investment   121

BOX 8.1

Seventh Foundational Principle of Population Health Science

Prevention of disease often yields a greater return on investment than curing disease after it has started.

---

health, over and above investment into treating disease. In the latter, we cannot take advantage of compounding and complementarity. This highlights our seventh principle of population health science, that prevention of disease has a greater ROI than curing disease after it starts (Box 8.1).

3.0 Assessing the Impact of Interventions over Time: Discounting Rates

The effects of short- versus long-term health benefits may or may not be compounded, but even if they are, they should be tempered with an evaluation of discounting rates. It is commonplace—although not without controversy (Torgerson and Raftery 1999)—to include discounting parameters into analyses of health investment return and other economic analyses of the cost-effectiveness of health interventions. The central idea behind discounting is to adjust the amount returned on a health intervention for inflation and other factors that influence the cost of spending a dollar now versus later. For example, suppose we have $10 to spend on a preventive intervention today. We could spend that money today or save the money and spend it 1 year from today. Two factors influence how much that $10 is worth 1 year from today. First, because of inflation, the value of each dollar may decrease. Second, if we invested the money in some way, the value of each dollar may increase. The difference between the inflationary decrease and the investment return increase is the discounting rate of the money. For example, if we could earn a 10% investment return but inflation is 3%, then the value of the $10 1 year from now is $10.70. Thus, if we spend $10 now rather than investing it, we are actually losing $10.70 during the course of 1 year. In sum, when spending money now, we must take into account not only the amount spent now, but the amount we would have accrued (investment return less inflation) if we had not spent it now.

Considering health returns on investment, however, the picture becomes more complicated, because what is the value of a healthy year now versus later, and what is a benefit of health now versus later? Such concepts exit the realm of pure econometrics and enter a more fuzzy discussion into the value of health for individuals and populations. For example, millions of sunburns occur each summer as beachgoers flock to their favorite sun spots, and future detriments to health in terms of skin cancers and other health problems result. However, the short-term enjoyment of a day at the beach produces many immediate benefits—relaxation, quality time with family, exercise, and enjoyment. Thus, an intervention to close all beaches to reduce the risk of future skin cancer would need to be discounted for the short-term consequence of reduced quality of life today. Furthermore, preventing someone from a day at the beach today does not, unlike money, produce a directly measurable investment return 1 year from now. Thus, the discounting rate of that day at the beach is difficult to quantify.

This "cost" of delaying an activity that is pleasurable today for a potential return tomorrow is often termed an *opportunity cost* or a *time preference*, and is difficult to qualify for most health-related outcomes. An early intervention to influence literacy levels, for example, may have long-lasting health and wellness benefits. Yet, forcing kids to be in the classroom takes away from activities they might enjoy more, such as playing outside. Thus, the return on teaching children to read 6 months earlier must be discounted by the outside playtime they missed during that process. As another example, consider the ROI of preventing binge drinking. It is intuitive that an intervention to prevent future binge drinking would have a greater return for health if we intervened at age 16 rather than age 50. However, there is an opportunity cost to such an intervention, because alcohol consumption is a pleasurable activity and many drinkers may prefer to have a year of binge drinking now even if it may cost them health-wise later. Thus, when considering the short-term and long-term return on health to the cost of preventing one case of binge drinking at age 16, the potential benefits of such an intervention could be tempered by the opportunity cost of not engaging in an activity that is pleasurable.

4.0 A Visual Description of the Relation Between Intervention and Return on Health

In Figure 8.1, we show the relationship between duration of disease and change in DALYs with and without an intervention for three models of

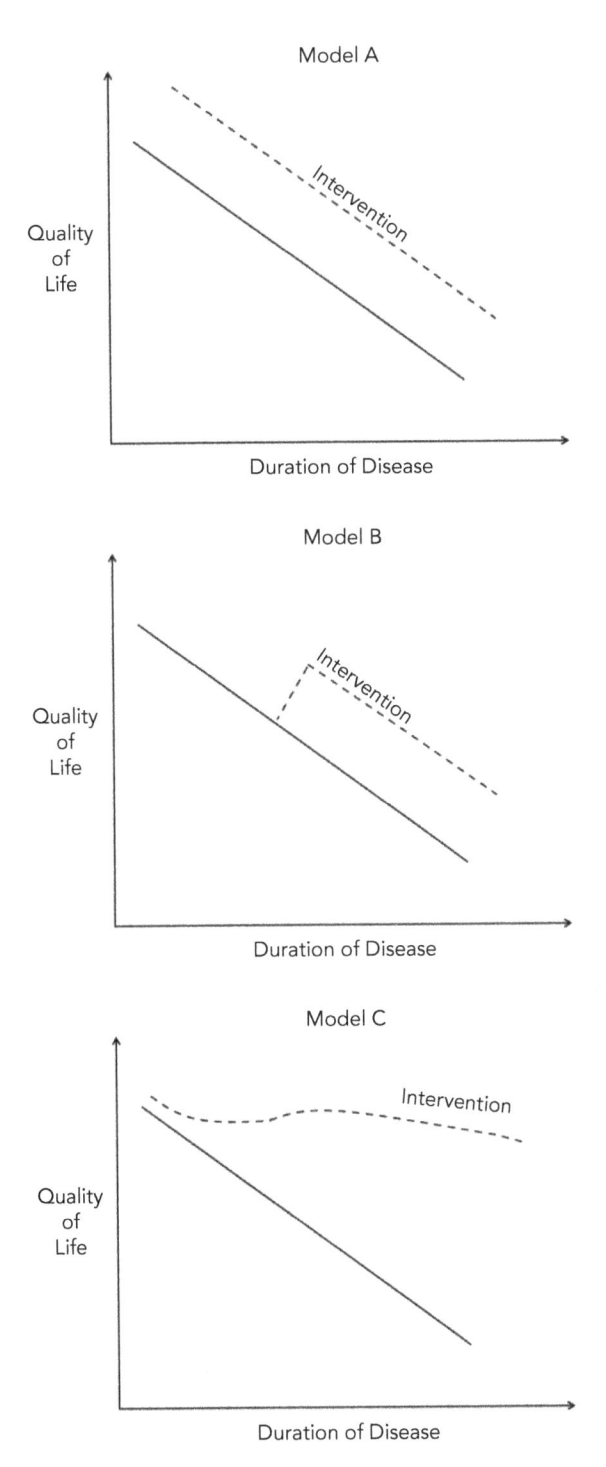

FIGURE 8.1 The relationship between duration of disease and change in disability-adjusted life years with and without an intervention for three models of intervention effects.

intervention effects. In model A, the intervention has a constant effect on change in DALYs. At the start of the intervention, those who are exposed have a reduction in the DALYs associated with the disease, and this reduction lasts throughout the duration of the disease. In model B, the intervention also has a constant effect on change in DALYs, but it has a lagged start such that the benefits of the intervention are not immediately apparent. In model C, the intervention has compounded returns. Not only does the intervention have an effect from the time of enactment among those exposed, but the improvement in DALYs magnifies throughout the duration of the disease. There are many other models that could be used to conceptualize how an intervention may influence the course of an illness; we chose these three for their clarity.

In summary of sections 3.0 and 4.0, when we evaluate the return on a dollar of investment today for health returns, we must consider a multitude of factors. The "interest" gained on that dollar may compound over time, with early investments having greater returns over time than later investments. However, there is a cost to such early investments in terms of opportunity time to engage in activities that might be pleasurable.

5.0 Hidden and Unintended Costs or Consequences

Matters are even more complicated than we have discussed thus far. When we conceptualize an end point for a certain intervention, there can be substantial costs (both in terms of money and in terms of health) that are hidden if we are not careful to realize and fully conceptualize all the ways in which our intervention can have an effect.

For example, suppose we have an intervention that has a high ROI for preventing stroke among individuals in their 60s and 70s. On average, we prevent about 10,000 strokes per year using this intervention, at a very low cost per stroke. We hail the intervention as a great public health success. However, although we may prevent stroke and its associated sequelae, those individuals who would have died of stroke are going to die eventually of other causes, and those other causes may be costly to treat and debilitating, and, potentially, the life of the individual who was prevented from having a stroke may not be prolonged substantially.

Thinking through the hidden health and other costs of public health interventions can be a difficult endeavor. For example, cigarette smoking is among the most preventable causes of death worldwide; it is attributed to more than 6 million deaths per year, and even more in chronic disease incidence and persistence (Centers for Disease Control and Prevention 2015, World Health Organization 2015). Preventing smoking would not only save millions of lives, but also would reduce health care expenditures by billions of dollars in the United States alone (Levy and Newhouse 2011). Ample evidence indicates there are both short- and long-term benefits of even small reductions in smoking prevalence at the population level, not only for population health but also for hospitalization and other health care costs, worker productivity, and many other metrics important to the overall functioning of a healthy society (Cummings et al. 1989, Parrott et al. 2000, Tsai et al. 2005, Barone-Adesi et al. 2006, Herman and Walsh 2011). However, there are hidden costs associated with reducing smoking. For example, millions of individuals living longer means there will be a greater strain on resources for elder care. These individuals may develop other illnesses common in old age that require substantial health care resources, long-term care facilities, caregiver services, and expensive treatment. A simulation study from 1997 indicated that, although there would be a short-term economic benefit if all smoking in the Netherlands were eliminated, health care costs would actually increase in the long term as a result of diseases incurred at older ages among those who would have died of smoking-related diseases (Barendregt et al. 1997). Simulation analyses of tobacco reduction programs indicate that Social Security resources in the United States would be compromised if all smokers quit, by increasing the percentage of people drawing on their Social Security benefits for a longer period of time, although that strain would be offset by increased productivity in the workforce as would-be smokers would work more and longer, and would be less affected by days missed as a result of disability (Hurd et al. 2011). Other potential consequences of smoking reduction may be effects on communities that rely on tobacco farming and other tobacco-related products for income, shortfalls in tax revenue in high-smoking areas, and other economic and social outcomes that may transform the structural ways in which revenue is generated in many communities. This change in revenue structure may have cascading effects on health, if unemployment increases and health care benefits are lost.

Of course, we do not suggest that public health programs to reduce smoking be abolished because it would be a strain on Social Security and we may not collect as much in taxes; however, thinking through the population level implications carefully in multiple sectors is part of the complicated calculations we face in population health science. If we endeavor to generate estimates of ROI in reducing smoking, we must contend with the morbid fact that all those would-be smokers will eventually die of something, and that "something" should be factored into the estimates on the returns to the health and economy of populations. More broadly, any attempt to estimate the ROI of a particular intervention should consider not only a particular health indicator of interest, but also the myriad potential consequences (both positive and negative) of a particular intervention.

6.0 Summary

Preventing disease often yields a greater ROI than curing disease after it has started. Documenting this ROI is critical to demonstrating the impact of population health approaches and building sustainable and durable support for these efforts. Challenges include deciding which return is of interest (e.g., reduced incidence, mortality, more productive years of life, more quality years of life) and evaluating the short- versus long-term benefits of interventions as well as unintended consequences. A focus on investment returns can demonstrate how preventive population health interventions, especially early during the life course, have the greatest possible potential to have long-term efficacy for population health production.

7.0 References

Barendregt, J. J., L. Bonneux, and P. J. van der Maas. (1997). The health care costs of smoking. *N Engl J Med* **337**(15): 1052–1057.

Barone-Adesi, F., L. Vizzini, F. Merletti, and L. Richiardi. (2006). Short-term effects of Italian smoking regulation on rates of hospital admission for acute myocardial infarction. *Eur Heart J* **28**(18): 2296.

Bruvold, W. H. (1993). A meta-analysis of adolescent smoking prevention programs. *Am J Public Health* **83**(6): 872–880.

Centers for Disease Control and Prevention. (2015). *Tobacco-related mortality*. Fact sheet. Accessed at http://www.cdc.gov/tobacco/data_statistics/fact_sheets/health_effects/tobacco_related_mortality/.

Cummings, S. R., S. M. Rubin, and G. Oster. (1989). The cost-effectiveness of counseling smokers to quit. *JAMA* **261**(1): 75–79.

Cunha, F., J. J. Heckman, and S. M. Schennach. (2010). Estimating the technology of cognitive and noncognitive skill formation. *Econometrica* **78**(3): 883–931.

Fanshel, S., and J. W. Bush. (1970). A health-status index and its application to health-services outcomes. *Oper Res* **18**(6): 1021–1066.

Heckman, J. J. (2000). Policies to foster human capital. *Res Econom* **54**(1): 3–56.

Heckman, J. J. (2006). Skill formation and the economics of investing in disadvantaged children. *Science* **312**(5782): 1900–1902.

Heckman, J. J. (2007). The economics, technology, and neuroscience of human capability formation. *Proc Natl Acad Sci U S A* **104**(33): 13250–13255.

Heckman, J. J. (2008). "Schools, skills, and synapses." *Econ Inq* **46**(3): 289–324.

Herman, P. M., and M. E. Walsh. (2011). Hospital admissions for acute myocardial infarction, angina, stroke, and asthma after implementation of Arizona's comprehensive statewide smoking ban. *Am J Public Health* **101**(3): 491–496.

Hurd, M., Y. Zheng, F. Girosi, and D. Goldman. (2011). The effects of tobacco control policy changes on the Social Security Trust Fund. In *After tobacco: what would happen if Americans stopped smoking?* P. Bearman, K. M. Neckerman, and L. Wright, editors. New York: Columbia University Press: 289–321.

Karoly, L. A., and H. P. Levaux. (1998). *Investing in our children: what we know and don't know about the costs and benefits of early childhood interventions.* Santa Monica, CA: Rand Corporation.

Lee, A., and R. Maheswaran. (2011). The health benefits of urban green spaces: a review of the evidence. *J Public Health* **33**(2): 212–222.

Levy, D. E., and J. P. Newhouse. (2011). Assessing the effects of tobacco policy changes on smoking-related health expenditures. In *After tobacco: what would happen if Americans stopped smoking?* P. Bearman, K. M. Neckerman, and L. Wright. New York: Columbia University Press: 256–289.

Parrott, S., C. Godfrey, and M. Raw. (2000). Costs of employee smoking in the workplace in Scotland. *Tob Control* **9**(2): 187–192.

Prieto, L., and J. A. Sacristan. (2003). Problems and solutions in calculating quality-adjusted life years (QALYs). *Health Qual Life Outcomes* **1**: 80–88.

Resch, S., E. Korenromp, J. Stover, M. Blakley, C. Krubiner, K. Thorien, et al. (2011). Economic returns to investment in AIDS treatment in low and middle income countries. *PLoS One* **6**(10): e25310.

Sassi, F. (2006). Calculating QALYs, comparing QALY and DALY calculations. *Health Policy Plann* **21**(5): 402–408.

Schweinhart, L. J., H. V. Barnes, and D. P. Weikart. (1993). *Significant benefits: the High/Scope Perry Preschool Study through age 27.* Ypsilanti, MI: High/Scope Press.

Tobler, N. S., M. R. Roona, P. Ochshorn, D. G. Marshall, A. V. Streke, and K. M. Stackpole. (2000). School-based adolescent drug prevention programs: 1998 meta-analysis. *J Prim Prev* **20**(4): 275–336.

Torgerson, D. J., and J. Raftery. (1999). Economic notes: discounting. *BMJ* **319**(7214): 914–915.

Torrance, G. W. (1970). *A generalized cost-effectiveness model for the evaluation of health programs.* Research report series 101. Hamilton, Faculty of Business, McMaster University.

Torrance, G. W., W. H. Thomas, and D. L. Sackett. (1972). A utility maximization model for evaluation of health care programs. *Health Serv Res* **7**(2): 118–133.

Tsai, S. P., C. P. Wen, S. C. Hu, T. Y. Cheng, and S. J. Huang. (2005). Workplace smoking related absenteeism and productivity costs in Taiwan. *Tob Control* **14**(Suppl 1): i33–i37.

Wilson, D., A. Kwon, J. Anderson, H. Thein, M. Law, L. Maher, G. Dore, and J. Kaldor. (2009). *Return on investment 2: evaluating the cost-effectiveness of needle and syringe programs in Australia.* Canberra; Australia: Publications Production Unit (Public Affairs, Parliamentary and Access Branch) Commonwealth Department of Health and Ageing.

World Health Organization. (2015). *Tobacco: fact sheet no. 339.* Retrieved from http://www.who.int/mediacentre/factsheets/fs339/en/.

Zeckhauser, R., and D. Shepard. (1976). Where now for saving lives? *Law Contemp Probl* 40: 5–45.

9

Equity and Efficiency in Population Health Science

WE HAVE, thus far in this book, focused on understanding population health science with the goal of improving the health of populations. We outlined how to think about populations, about population health, about its causes, and about how to weight the various causes of population health so we may intervene to maximize the health of populations. However, this discussion has elided one core part of our definition of population health science, as offered in Chapter 1: the distributions of health within populations or, put simply, the health gaps or health inequalities that characterize the health of populations worldwide.

Health inequities are deeply embedded within populations. Groups with power, prestige, and resources have better health than those who do not have such status (Link and Phelan, 1994). These inequalities are not idiosyncratic "differences" across groups, but arise as a result of the distribution of resources in a way that privileges those with more status. Therefore, inequalities in health refer to differences generated by social and political structures, and can be undone (i.e., are not immutable). From the seminal publication of the Whitehall studies in 1978 (Marmot et al. 1978), the Black report in 1980 (Department of Health and Social Security 1980), and throughout the past three decades (Glymour et al. 2014), inequalities in health by socioeconomic class that are not explainable by social selection or other methodological artifacts have been at the forefront of a movement in population health to confront the drivers of sickness and disease at a structural level.

The terms *inequity* and *inequality*—the two words that have common currency in population health science—have very specific meanings. *Inequality* typically refers to a *difference*, and the two words are often used interchangeably.

Inequity, as used in population health science, suggests the difference observed between groups is a result of a process rooted in injustice and unfair treatment (e.g., experiences of discrimination differ between blacks and whites). Therefore, a difference between two groups can be considered to be an *inequality* without being *inequitable* if it is a result of biological or other social factors that are not fundamentally unjust (e.g., women are more likely to have breast cancer than men, not because of a social injustice but because of their biology). Somewhat confusingly, inequity and inequality are used differently in various disciplines (and sometimes within disciplines), and we use examples from various intellectual traditions in this chapter. For the purposes of this chapter, then, we use the following definitions: *inequality* refers to a quantitative difference between outcomes for groups; *inequity* refers to an inequality that is unfair, stemming from an unjust distribution of resources.

This chapter tackles two concepts—equity and efficiency—both of which are important for population health science, and are inextricably linked to inequalities in several ways. Efficiency pertains to the potential success we may have in implementing efforts to improve population health, or maximizing the greatest ROI for the greatest number of people. At a fundamental level, we in population health science should endeavor to create and implement policies and programs that maximize the amount of health in a population. Ruthless maximization of a population's total potential for health makes for efficient interventions.

When considering initiatives—both those aimed at shifting the curve of population health as well as those aimed at high-risk groups—ideally, we want population health interventions that are both efficient and equitable. In many ways, however, these two goals—equity and efficiency—are often at odds with each other; that is, there is a tradeoff when maximizing one potentially results in a cost for the other. We note this is not true in all circumstances, and many programs are distributed both efficiently and equitably (Reidpath et al. 2012). However, careful consideration of the potential for inefficiency and inequality, especially in how improving efficiency may affect inequality, remains an important tenet of promoting a population health system that aligns with our values.

This chapter is divided into four parts. First, we discuss definitions and offer examples of equity and efficiency deriving from several bodies of literature. Second, we provide some examples from population health science of when equity and efficiency are in conflict, and potential resolutions of those conflicts. Third, we present examples when equity and efficiency are not in conflict, and how this informs our general understanding of these concepts. Finally, we provide an overview of how to integrate these concepts into our value system as population health scientists.

1.0 What Are Equity and Efficiency?

The concepts of equity and efficiency are foundational to economic science and are used in a wide variety of other disciplines. Because these terms are applied in a wide variety of contexts, there is tremendous variation in the definitions used for both equity and efficiency, the way in which they are applied, and the types of situations that are considered (Culyer and Wagstaff 1993). For our purposes, we use definitions and examples we find to be most helpful in the context of population health science, while acknowledging that other definitions could be used and other conclusions could be drawn from our examples given a different set of starting assumptions.

In economics, efficiency is referred to as the maximization of the total economic output of a system, and equity as the extent to which there is even distribution of those outputs. There are several classic examples of these two concepts in the economics literature (Le Grand 1990). For example, paraphrasing an example by Le Grand (1990), government welfare programs often aim to increase equity because they redistribute wealth from those with the most to those with the least, but they may be inefficient if they produce disincentives from productive labor market participation. Alternatively, a fixed tax amount on all residents in the United States is highly efficient; there is low disincentive to continue to be productive in the labor market because the tax is due regardless of whether an individual works, but it is highly inequitable because billionaires owe the same tax as those struggling to survive. In both these examples, there is a tradeoff between efficiency and equity. The more evenly we distribute wealth, the (theoretically) less efficient the marketplace of labor will be; in the same regard, the more we have an efficient tax system for maximization of the labor marketplace, the less equitable the distribution of those taxes will be.

These examples from economics make clear that much of the discussion about equity and efficiency refers to what we value most in terms of the type of society we want to create. Some societies have higher thresholds for equitable distribution of wealth and resources; others find the idea of equity to be antithetical to ideals of personal liberty and agency. Consider, for example, the concept of Pareto efficiency. A system is Pareto efficient when there can be no change that would improve one person's situation without worsening anther person's situation. Having Pareto efficiency is considered to be a desirable economic condition for a system in terms of efficiency under certain assumptions

(Newbery and Stiglitz 1984). Although the concept that no one is able to be better off without making someone worse off seems as if it would correlate with equity, it, in fact, does not because there are many ways to make a system Pareto efficient. If there is a total of $100 in the economy and five people, it is equally Pareto efficient to give each person $20 dollars or to give four people $25 and one person nothing. In the former case, we are clearly both Pareto efficient while being completely equitable; in the latter case, we are Pareto efficient, because no one can be made better off without affecting someone else adversely, but we are not equitable. Thus, which Pareto-efficient outcome we want depends on whether we value everyone having the same amount or whether some having the most and some having the least is acceptable.

2.0 Equity and Efficiency in Population Health

When we move from the economic definitions to the applications of equity and efficiency in health systems, we change the frame from maximizing the total productive output (e.g., amount of money generated) of a population to maximizing the total health of a population. That is, we seek to maximize the "health output" of the population, including minimizing DALYs lost as a result of major acute and chronic conditions, extending years of productive life, and improving QALYs for those with serious disabilities and conditions (We introduced both DALYs and QALYs in Chapter 8). Furthermore, we want to improve health equitably—that is, we do not want those who are richest or those with the most resources to be the healthiest in a society that values health for all people.

It is this latter point that creates the core tension of interest. If we are interested in equity, it is unlikely to serve our purposes to take the total number of health dollars available in the economy and divide it up equally for everyone in the system. Using health care systems as an illustration, healthy people do not need the same number of health care dollars as sick people. How we decide to maximize efforts to achieve efficiency (the total health of the population) with equity speaks fundamentally to our core values as a society and how we treat those who are the least well off.

We can aspire to achieve equity in health through horizontal and vertical approaches. Horizontal equity refers to the distribution of health care resources according to need—those with the same level of need should get the same level of service in a horizontally equitable health system (Culyer and Wagstaff 1993, James et al. 2005). For example, two individuals who have an equal number of symptoms of disease should get an equal number of health care dollars and

Equity and Efficiency in Population Health Science 133

the same amount of health care quality. Vertical equity refers to focusing on expenditures (either in money or in labor) that increase the maximization of health capacity for those who need it most. For example, those who are the most sick should get the most services compared with those who are moderately sick. Both these concepts suggest we strive to both treat all those with the same level of sickness with the same level of services, and we attempt to distribute these services in a way that privileges those who need them most.

However, these efforts at equity in health care distribution, both horizontally and vertically, tangle with our desire to maximize efficiency. Efficiency in the population health context can be conceived in many ways, including total amount of years of life gained or reduction in disease incidence, but also may be considered in terms of return on health investment or cost-effectiveness per life saved. This tension becomes readily apparent when we consider the implications of universal health interventions—that is, efforts to improve health by delivering an intervention to all people. These interventions are often popular as a result of the perception that if an intervention is universal, it promotes equity because exposure is ubiquitous. And yet, universal interventions, even when very effective, can both create and exacerbate inequality.

For example, suppose we have two individuals, one who has a permanent physical disability and one who does not (Figure 9.1) (paraphrasing

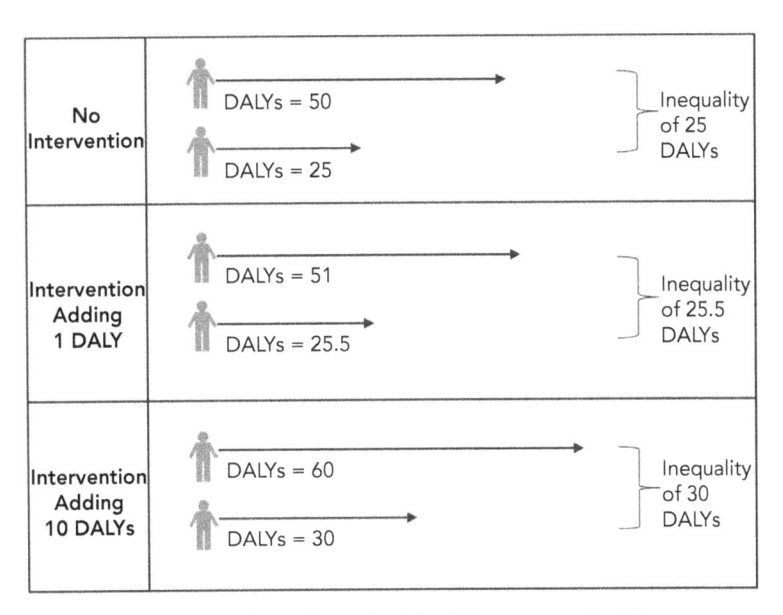

No Intervention	DALYs = 50 DALYs = 25	Inequality of 25 DALYs
Intervention Adding 1 DALY	DALYs = 51 DALYs = 25.5	Inequality of 25.5 DALYs
Intervention Adding 10 DALYs	DALYs = 60 DALYs = 30	Inequality of 30 DALYs

FIGURE 9.1 Gaining overall population health while increasing health inequity. DALY, disability-adjusted life year.

an example in Anand and Hanson [1998]). The person with a disability has a QALY weight of 0.5 (see Chapter 8 for a discussion of QALY weights), whereas the other person has a QALY weight of 1. If an intervention increases each of their lives by a year (DALY = 1), this net effect of this is to exacerbate the inequality in quality of life between the person with disabilities and the person without, because the effect of the 1 year gain for the person with disabilities is only half that of the person without. Thus, although increasing the DALYs for an entire population by 1 year may seem like a worthwhile public health goal, we must understand that the net effect of that goal may be to exacerbate inequality in factors that influence quality of life and other factors, which has to do with how that DALY is increased within the population.

As another example, suppose we are evaluating the potential return on health investment of a particular neighborhood intervention to improve the quality of life for individuals with a disabling chronic disease (Figure 9.2). The number of DALYs gained from the intervention will vary according to parameters associated with equity. Capacity to make life adjustments for a disabling chronic disease is more difficult among those with low resources; thus, the disability-adjusted weights for QALY and DALY estimation vary by factors such as socioeconomic status. The net effect of such an intervention may be to exacerbate differences between the wealthy and the poor, if

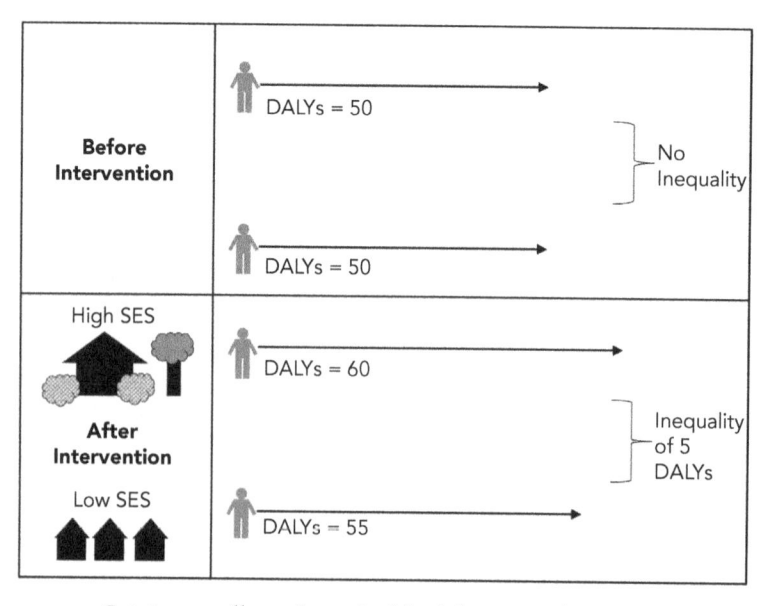

FIGURE 9.2 Gaining overall population health while creating health inequalities. DALY, disability-adjusted life year; SES, socioeconomic status.

those who are wealthy have a greater capacity to take advantage of a neighborhood intervention. Such considerations are well documented in sociological research on the emergence and persistence of health inequities; substantial research has documented that new information and technology in the marketplace related to health benefits those with the most resources first (Link and Phelan 1994, Phelan et al. 2004).

Finally, as a counterexample, let us consider the example of palliative care. Palliative care at the end of life is a quite equitable delivery of health care. Those at the end of life are often sickest and, per our vertical equity principles, those who are sickest should get the most resources. However, end-of-life care is not only expensive, but there is also often little total population health benefit in terms of years of life gained through palliative care. Yet, our value system as a society appreciates compassionate and quality end-of-life care for all over the lack of technical efficiency in palliative care.

Thus, although equity and efficiency are often considered to be tradeoffs of each other, in many circumstances they are causally related; universal interventions that are highly efficient may in turn create inequities that were not there previously. Understanding the impact of efficiency on equity is critical for evaluating the efficacy of a particular policy, program, or intervention, and the potential for unintended consequences, especially for vulnerable subgroups.

3.0 Equity and Efficiency in Population Health Science: Hypothetical and Empirical Examples

To understand the concept of equity versus efficiency in population health, imagine we have two hypothetical interventions to improve population health. Both interventions cost the same amount of money, but we do not have enough resources to operationalize both. Furthermore, both interventions have the same impact on population it terms of pure efficiency parameters, such as total years of life gained. Suppose that with intervention 1, we can increase the length of life for 50 individuals by 2 years. With intervention 2, we can increase the length of life for 100 individuals by 1 year. Thus, with no additional information we would assume that, in aggregate, we are gaining 100 person-years of life through either intervention. We need to decide, as population health scientists, whether to recommend intervention 1 or intervention 2.

In terms of total efficiency, as measured by years of life gained, these interventions are equally beneficial for society. We may want to examine other metrics as well, such as productive years of life in the labor force, should that be something we value (it may not). Thus, if the 100 years of life gained with intervention 1 are all for individuals older than 90 years whereas the 100 years of life gained with intervention 2 are all for individuals younger than 30, we may, in pure efficiency parameters, privilege intervention 2 because we will have more economic and other output from those years compared with an individual at the end of life. As noted, however, this creates inequity, because we are valuing a young life more than an older life, thus we are making a value judgment about the good to society of an additional year of life at different ages.

Furthermore, we may want to consider other equity parameters when deciding between these two interventions. Are we creating or maintaining inequality with respect to socioeconomic status or other marginalized social statuses with either intervention? Is the delivery of the intervention and the process through which each intervention is implemented equitable horizontally and vertically? If not, which intervention is likely to have the greatest impact on generating or maintaining inequities?

In summary, although some have tried to place a numerical value on the cost of a year of life while remaining unbiased to whom the year of life is given, equity considerations across subgroups suggest that a wide range of value-laden assumptions need to be made to engage with conclusions about the economic or noneconomic value of a year of life gained (Wagstaff 1991), and also that equity considerations should be given to the value of years of life gained or quality of life gained to reduce health inequality (Cookson et al. 2009).

Interventions during early childhood for long-term prevention are often highly efficient—more efficient than preventive interventions later in life. From a sheer efficiency standpoint, the number of years of productivity to society from saving a child's life is likely greater than saving the life of an older adult. Plus, there are benefits to early-childhood intervention beyond mortality. For example, for obese adults, it would have been much more cost-effective to prevent obesity from occurring through interventions in childhood than reducing weight among those who are already obese. Preventing disease in childhood has the capacity to have the maximum impact on years of life saved, and may have positive unintended consequences for other outcomes (Heckman 2006, Heckman 2007). Yet, investing more resources in saving a child's life than an older adult is not equitable. Imagine two individuals with the same condition, one acquiring the condition during childhood and one during adulthood. Under the definition of horizontal equity, these two individuals should get the same resources. Investing more in child health rather than adult health privileges efficiency at the expense of equity. There are examples of this in the literature. For example, among individuals in need of a kidney transplant, younger age is privileged when two individuals meet the same criteria based on medical need (Ladin and Hanto 2011), under the assumptions that more DALYs will be saved by transplanting the kidney to a younger person than an older person. Many have criticized such parameters as an age-based discriminatory practice, indicating that the efficiency we might gain must be balanced by the equity in valuing life no matter the age. As stated throughout this chapter, we may accept some inequity to maximize efficiency, and the level of inequity that we as a society are willing to accept is an important parameter to estimate when determining the ideal balance between the two.

4.0 When Equity and Efficiency Are Not in Conflict

Although equity and efficiency are often considered to be tradeoffs, it is not a universal truth that we must abandon one for the other. There are certainly examples in the health literature when equity and efficiency are aligned, and these types of interventions are often beneficial for public health.

Consider, for example, screening programs to detect the presence of treatable illness. We can either screen universally or focus on screening groups that are at particular risk for disease. If we screen universally, we may miss cases of disease in the high-risk groups because we are focused on delivering the intervention to all and accepting some noncompliance. If we focus instead on maximizing compliance in the hard-to-reach group, we may be able to detect more cases. Furthermore, screening universally is not necessarily equitable. Although all individuals have the same access to the service, horizontal equity suggests those with the same level of need are provided with the same level of service, and if risk of disease varies across groups, then there is not a need for universal screening. Thus, high-risk screening is often both equitable and efficient.

Equity–efficiency tradeoffs have been discussed in the literature with respect to sickle cell anemia, which can be screened for and is more likely to affect particular racial/ethnic minority groups (Sassi et al. 2001). Screening for sickle cell anemia universally is neither cost-effective nor efficient, nor equitable per the principles discussed earlier. Although all individuals get the same intervention (screening), inequity could be exacerbated because cases in hard-to-reach groups are missed, and universal screening may violate the principle of providing equal services to those in equal need. Other screening examples in which equity and efficiency are not in conflict include screening for lung cancer. Limiting screening to smokers is both efficient (because smokers are the most likely to develop lung cancer) and equitable (because the burden of lung cancer in smokers is much greater than in nonsmokers).

5.0 Our Value System as Population Health Scientists

Theoretically, it is our responsibility as population health scientists to improve the overall population's health. We may want to dive headfirst into that endeavor, ruthlessly pursuing efficiency and maximization of years of live saved. But such pursuit is not always optimal; we may create, maintain, or exacerbate inequities in population health if efficiency is prioritized over equity. This highlights our eighth foundational principle of population health science (Box 9.1).

Evaluation of the relationship between equity and efficiency is critical to a functioning population health science that seeks to maximize health. Although equity and efficiency are often referred to in terms of a tradeoff, both are about the process through which interventions and other services are delivered, rather than the outcome of those processes, and thus are not always inherently in conflict. In fact, equity and efficiency are in conflict only to the extent they are dependent on the outcome or output of interest. Interventions can be both equitable and efficient, but the relevant questions are "Who deems the equity has been achieved?" and "What is the process through which efficiency was determined?" Because the same intervention can have numerous interpretations for various outcomes, and there is a cost tradeoff when an intervention that is more equitable and more efficient could have been overlooked, the evaluation of equity and efficiency is often in the eye of the beholder.

The optimal balance between equity and efficiency cannot be determined solely by quantitative analysis. The optimal balance depends on our values and goals as a society, and maximizing them within the reality of a limited

---

BOX 9.1

Eighth Foundational Principle of Population Health Science

Efforts to improve overall population health may be a disadvantage to some groups; whether equity or efficiency is preferable is a matter of values.

and finite pool of resources. As an example, consider the discussions around health care reform in the United States in 2012. A hot-button issue during the 2012 election, for example, included provisions regarding the use of committee decisions for allocation of health care resources among those with low survival probability. For example, the public seemingly recoiled at the idea that bureaucrats were going to decide on the continuation of services for those close to death based on cost of services. Similar provisions have been enacted, albeit not without controversy, in several other countries with national health services. The debate reveals the conflict between equity and efficiency. There is a maximum number of dollars that can be spent on health and health care, and we need to decide how best to use those resources efficiently. One way in which to do this is to prioritize those cases in which the potential additional DALYs and QALYs are the highest per dollar spent; however, this means our sickest individuals may not get the maximum amount of care that could be given to increase their life by an additional year or to improve their quality of life in the most optimal way. However, pure equality across age in health care resources is inefficient, depending on what outcome we consider to be most important (e.g., productive years of life that can be spent in the labor force). Thus, the answer to the question of how to distribute these resources depends on what we value and how we value it, and the political and social will to create a system that reflects these shared valuations.

Ultimately, evaluations of equity and efficiency tradeoffs are much like everything else in population health: their quantitative and qualitative evaluation depends on a set of values and goals. Population health scientists have a moral obligation to address inequalities as they arise from inequities in the distribution of resources. Such obligation necessitates entanglement with considerations about whether proposed interventions will result in widening equity gaps at the expense of efficiency. Understanding who sets the goals and whether those goals are optimal for maximizing population health remains, perhaps, the most important job of a population health scientist.

6.0 References

Anand, S., and K. Hanson. (1998). DALYs: efficiency versus equity. *World Dev* **26**(2): 307–310.

Cookson, R., M. Drummond, and H. Weatherly. (2009). Explicit incorporation of equity considerations into economic evaluation of public health interventions. *Health Econ Policy Law* **4**(2): 231–245.

Culyer, A. J., and A. Wagstaff. (1993). Equity and equality in health and health care. *J Health Econ* **12**: 431–457.

Department of Health and Social Security. (1980). *Inequalities in health: report of a research working group*. London: Department of Health and Social Security.

Glymour, M., M. Avendano, and I. Kawachi. (2014). Socioeconomic status and health. In *Social epidemiology* (2nd edition). L. Berkman, I. Kawachi, and M. Glymour, editors. New York: Oxford University Press: 17–62.

Heckman, J. J. (2006). Skill formation and the economics of investing in disadvantaged children. *Science* **312**(5782): 1900–1902.

Heckman, J. J. (2007). The economics, technology, and neuroscience of human capability formation. *Proc Natl Acad Sci U S A* **104**(33): 13250–13255.

James, C., G. Carrin, W. Savedoff, and P. Hanvoravongchai. (2005). Clarifying efficiency–equity tradeoffs through explicit criteria, with a focus on developing countries. *Health Care Anal* **13**(1): 33–51.

Ladin, K., and D. W. Hanto. (2011). Rational rationing or discrimination: balancing equity and efficiency considerations in kidney allocation. *Am J Transplant* **11**(11): 2317–2321.

Le Grand, J. (1990). Equity versus efficiency: the elusive trade-off. *Ethics* **100**(3): 554–568.

Link, B. G., and J. Phelan. (1994). Social conditions as fundamental causes of disease. *J Health Soc Behav* **35**: 80–94.

Marmot, M. G., G. Rose, M. Shipley, and P. J. Hamilton. (1978). Employment grade and coronary heart disease in British civil servants. *J Epidemiol Commun Health* **32**(4): 244–249.

Newbery, D. M. G., and J. E. Stiglitz. (1984). Pareto inferior trade. *Rev Econ Stud* **51**(1): 1–12.

Phelan, J., B. G. Link, A. Diez-Roux, I. Kawachi, and B. Levin. (2004). 'Fundamental causes' of social inequalities in mortality: a test of the theory. *J Health Soc Behav* **45**(3): 265–285.

Reidpath, D. D., A. E. Olafsdottir, S. Pokhrel, and P. Allotey. (2012). The fallacy of the equity–efficiency trade off: rethinking the efficient health system. *BMC Public Health* **12**: S3.

Sassi, F., J. Le Grand, and L. Archard. (2001). Equity versus efficiency: a dilemma for the NHS. *BMJ* **323**: 762–763.

Wagstaff, A. (1991). QALYs and the equity–efficiency trade-off. *J Health Econ* **10**: 21–41.

10

Prediction in Population Health Science

ONE OF THE key challenges faced by population health is the intuitive way in which we—as both researchers and potential patients—rely on individual experiences for data on health. As discussed in previous chapters, our approach to health tends to focus on our own individual health—that is: What makes me healthy? Such endeavors have become increasingly popular in the health sciences. For example, "predictive" and "personalized" medicine are major efforts across a variety of domains to transfer knowledge from epidemiological and clinical science to meaningful treatments and preventive efforts aimed at the individual rather than the group (Collins and McKusick 2001, Hamburg and Collins 2010, Collins and Varmus 2015). Much of the investment in this effort has been in identifying individuals with particular genotypes that place them at higher risk for disease outcomes (Smith 2011, Wray et al. 2013, Bayer and Galea 2015).

The concerns of population health are different. Population health is concerned with disease occurrence, distributions, and causes according to averages. Rather than asking why a particular person became ill, we ask why certain populations have more or less burden of disease. Although conceptualizing disease according to averages is central to population health science, many clinicians, consumers, and stakeholders want to know how likely it is that a certain person will develop or not develop a specific illness based on the average across individuals. To know how likely an individual is to develop a

---

Note: Portions of the text in this chapter are adapted from: Keyes, K. M., G. Davey Smith, K. Koenen, and S. Galea. (2015). "The mathematical limits of genetic prediction for complex chronic disease." *J Epidemiol Commun Health* ePub February 3. http://www.ncbi.nlm.nih.gov/pubmed/25648993

certain health indicator based on a certain risk factor or set of risk factors, we need to know how to transfer the average measures of association we obtain from population health studies to prediction, and test how well our predictions perform in real-world settings.

Key questions remain about whether an individualized, predictive approach is likely to yield meaningful change at the population level in relation to the health indicators that are most pervasive. A central issue is how well predictive measures can judge whether an individual will develop an outcome of interest and, subsequently, what we can do about the outcome of interest in the face of a solid predictive measure.

In this chapter we review fundamental methods for assessing predictive validity through positive predictive value, discuss the limitations of translating population measures to individualized prediction, and provide an example highlighting the limitations of predictive individual approaches for population health.

1.0 Assessing Predictive Validity: Positive Predictive Value

Prediction uses estimated measures that correlate with an outcome to make a probabilistic guess about what will happen in the future. We predict whether it is going to rain tomorrow using what is known about geography, wind patterns, temperature, and a host of other factors correlated with particular weather events. Although such predictive models for weather are generally quite sophisticated, all of us have had the experience of bringing our umbrella to work because of the prediction of rain, only to find the sun shines all day, without a cloud in the sky. Predicting health events based on correlated factors is quite similar, albeit based on evidence that is often not as well tested.

Although predictive validity models can take many forms, the most basic estimate is the positive predictive validity of a measure or set of measures. To describe positive predictive validity, consider the following example. Suppose we are interested in estimating whether we can predict who will develop heart disease in adulthood based on childhood socioeconomic status indicators such as parental education and housing conditions. Such questions are based on the life course and multilevel models of population health described in previous chapters. In general, it is found that children living in impoverished conditions develop heart disease at about 1.5 to 2.0 times the rate of those who do not (Smith et al. 1998, Lawlor et al. 2004). We might conclude, then, that childhood poverty is an important risk factor for adult disease.

However, such a conclusion based on rate ratios or other measures of association do not tell us how predictive childhood poverty is for the development of heart disease. Rather, we need to ask the question in a different way—for example: Given that a certain individual was born in impoverished conditions, what is the probability he or she will develop heart disease by age 65?

To answer this question, we can estimate the positive predictive value of childhood poverty. Table 10.1 includes a two-by-two contingency table of hypothetical data for childhood poverty and development of heart disease by age 65, and the risk ratio for the association between childhood poverty and heart disease, estimated by dividing the risk of heart disease among those with childhood poverty by the risk of heart disease among those without childhood poverty.

$$\text{Risk Ratio} : \frac{\left(\frac{25}{200}\right)}{\left(\frac{50}{800}\right)} = 2.0.$$

As seen by the previous equation, the risk of heart disease by age 65 among those with childhood poverty is 2.0 times that of those without childhood poverty.

However, let us look at the positive predictive value, which is the conditional probability of disease given that individuals are in the childhood poverty group:

$$\text{Positive Predictive Value} = \frac{25}{200} = 0.125 \text{ or } 12.5\%.$$

Thus, although childhood poverty is a robust risk factor for heart disease, the vast majority of individuals with childhood poverty do not develop heart disease according to these data. Using childhood poverty as a predictive factor for who will develop heart disease is not advisable in this case.

Table 10.1 Population 1: Childhood Poverty as a Risk Factor for Adult Heart Disease by Age 65 Years in a Population of 1000 Individuals

Presence of Childhood Poverty	Heart Disease	No Heart Disease	Total
Childhood poverty	25	175	200
No childhood poverty	50	750	800
Total	100	900	1000

Conversely, we could also examine the negative predictive value. Given that an individual did not experience poverty as a child, what is the probability he or she does not develop heart disease?

$$\text{Negative Predictive Value} = \frac{75}{800} = 0.9375 \text{ or } 93.8\%.$$

We see the negative predictive value is much greater than the positive predictive value. In this example, if an individual experiences childhood poverty there is a 12.5% probability of developing heart disease by age 65, but if he or she did not experience childhood poverty, there is a 93.8% probability he or she will not develop heart disease.

In contrast, consider another population (population 2), with the same exposure of interest (childhood poverty), presented in Table 10.2, as well as the risk ratio for the association between childhood poverty and heart disease.

$$\text{Risk Ratio} = \frac{\frac{100}{200}}{\frac{200}{800}} = 2.0.$$

We see that population 2 has the same number of individuals (1000), the same prevalence of childhood poverty (200/1000, or 20%), and the same risk ratio for the association between childhood poverty and heart disease by age 65. But now let us examine the positive predictive value:

$$\text{Positive Predictive Value} = \frac{100}{200} = 0.50 \text{ or } 50\%.$$

From population 1 to population 2, we have the same strength of association between the exposure and the outcome based on the risk ratio, but the

Table 10.2 Population 2: Childhood Poverty as a Risk Factor for Adult Heart Disease by Age 65 Years in a Population of 1000 Individuals

Presence of Childhood Poverty	Heart Disease	No Heart Disease	Total
Childhood poverty	100	100	200
No childhood poverty	200	600	800
Total	300	700	1000

predictive value of the exposure is much greater. Now there is a 50% probability an individual with childhood poverty will develop heart disease, whereas in population 1 there was a 12.5% probability.

The negative predictive value, in turn, decreases from population 1 to population 2:

$$\text{Negative Predictive Value} = \frac{600}{800} = 0.75 \text{ or } 75\%.$$

The reason the predictive value increases so substantially from population 1 to population 2 is that the prevalence of heart disease increases: from 10% in population 1 to 30% in population 2. This underlies the fundamental concepts in using risk factors—regardless of whether they are genetic variants, clinical indicators, or social processes—to predict disease: the predictability is a function of the strength of the association between the indicator and the outcome as well as the prevalence of the outcome in the population of interest.

Such concepts are well known in the science of screening for disease; it is understood that even a highly valid screening measure should be applied to populations at high risk for disease to have a screening program that has a demonstrable impact on population health. In preventive medicine, predictive values have been used to assess outcomes such as stroke and heart disease, using risk score measures that take into account many known correlates (Wolf et al. 1991, Wilson et al. 1998, D'Agostino et al. 2001), such as the Framingham Risk Score, with varying degrees of predictability depending on the distributions of risk factors in the populations studied.

The variation in the predictability of a risk score based on characteristics of the population underlies the central concepts of interaction in the assessment of prediction, which are detailed later in this chapter in the example.

2.0 Limitations of Translating Population Measures to Individualized Prediction

Although assessing the positive predictive value of a risk factor or set of risk factors is an important part of assessing utility for preventive medicine in populations, the promise of individualized prediction for population health science faces some fundamental limitations. Importantly, a risk factor must be of strong magnitude to result in good prediction. Pepe et al. (2004) found that odds ratios, for example, need to have very high magnitudes to have predictive power. Even exposure–outcome relations with odds ratios as high as 3.0 have poor predictive power, and those in magnitudes of 10 to 20 are not optimal for predicting individualized disease risk. It is quite rare in population health, especially for those exposures with distal or diffuse effects, to have such strong magnitudes of risk. Furthermore, exposures with low magnitudes of risk may have strong predictive power when the outcomes they are predicting are prevalent or when the exposures themselves are highly prevalent.

The ongoing quest to create individualized estimates of disease risk based on factors such as genotypes highlights some limitations of prediction in population health. Single genetic variants rarely have strong enough associations to provide robust estimates of risk, and although polygenetic risk scores increase the predictive power of genotype-based prediction, the positive predictive values remain underwhelming for accurate prediction. There are, however, exceptions to such generalizations, albeit rare. For example, genetic variants in Leber hereditary optic neuropathy have a strong effect (clinical penetrance of >90%) among individuals who smoke (Kirkman et al. 2009). In a smoking population, those who have the risk gene almost inevitably develop the disease, whereas those who do not have the risk gene do not, which demonstrates the large effect of the gene. The predictability of Leber hereditary optic neuropathy would be close to perfect among populations of smokers. If smoking is not considered, the overall gene–disease association estimate is modest and the gene has less predictability on the outcome.

Further, individualized prediction within populations is fundamentally limited because of the principles outlined earlier in this book. We have demonstrated that factors that cause variation within populations may not be the same as factors that cause disease across populations, and to understand how population health manifests, we must conceptualize it as a continuum and consider the macro-, micro-, and life course factors that interact with each other within and across populations to cause distributions of health to occur.

3.0 Example: The Limits of Predictive Medicine for Population Health

As noted earlier, investment in understanding the genetic basis of human disease has long promised a potentially revolutionary way to predict which healthy individuals eventually develop disease (Collins and McKusick 2001, Hamburg and Collins 2010). Scholarly commentaries and the scientific lay media suggest the time is soon coming when the neighborhood general practitioner will scan patients' biological information to facilitate preventive recommendations (Hood and Flores 2012, Eisenberg 2013). Furthermore, an increasingly lucrative private industry promises to provide individuals with a prediction about their risk of disease based on their genetic profile (Prainsack et al. 2008, Wright and Gregory-Jones 2010, Bellcross et al. 2012). For secondary and tertiary prevention, the rapid advances in technology to scan the genome have brought important advances in identification and treatment of disease. In the case of pharmacogenetics, a relatively small but expanding range of established findings allows incorporation of germline genetic information to predict adverse events and drug response (Ong et al. 2012).

However, primary prevention based on common germline genetic variants has not, generally speaking, been successful (Janssens and van Duijn 2008, Davey Smith 2011, Voight et al. 2012, Wray et al. 2013). Large-scale genome-wide association studies have demonstrated that many chronic diseases are highly polygenic, with hundreds of genes explaining only a small portion of variance (Manolio et al. 2009, Major Depressive Disorder Working Group of the Psychiatric Genome-Wide Association Studies (GWAS) Consortium. 2013), obviating the utility of any one genetic factor (or a small set) in disease prediction. Certainly, the science and scholarship behind systems biology and genetic medicine is advancing rapidly (Hood and Flores 2012, Khoury et al. 2012), foreshadowing a potential future in which enough data points are available on enough biological systems within and across people that our current approaches to developing predictive tools may yield successful clinical utility.

Understanding the factors that may elicit genetic risk are critical to interpreting the magnitude of the effect (Rothman et al. 2008, Luo et al. 2013) because the magnitude of an association differs across populations with different distributions of other risk factors (Khoury et al. 2012). This understanding rests on concepts of interaction and of disease risk differing within and across populations. Here we demonstrate the utility of such concepts using a simulation approach.

3.1 Causal Structure of Disease

We begin our simulation by creating a causal structure for a hypothetical disease. In this hypothetical scenario, disease is caused through the interaction of a germline genetic risk variant and an environmental exposure (or a set of adverse environmental exposures). Individuals exposed to the genetic risk variant and the environmental exposure will have a higher risk of disease than the additive effect of those exposed to either factor alone (we note this is a more conservative assumption than an effect assumed to be interactive multiplicatively; the results of the simulation hold under assumptions of additive or multiplicative risk). The disease can also be caused in a myriad of other ways (i.e., unrelated to the genetic and environmental factor of central interest), which is represented in our simulation as the background rate of disease. Therefore, any increase in the risk of disease among those with the genetic variant is a relative increase over the background rate.

There are three parameters that are varied in our simulation: the prevalence of the genetic risk variant, the prevalence of the environmental context, and the background rate. For the purposes of this simulation, we denote the genetic variant as G, the environmental context of interest as E, and alternative causes as X. Therefore, in this example we are interested primarily in understanding how the risk ratio describing the association between G and disease varies at different values of E and X.

We note that the simulation we conduct is agnostic to what we define G and E to be. The simulation would be equally as accurate if, instead of an environmental factor, we posited a second genetic factor (epistasis). For simplicity, we focus on labeling the second factor as an environmental factor.

3.2 Simulated Populations

To estimate every conceivable combination of prevalence (from 1–100) for three factors, we needed to simulate 100 × 100 × 100 populations (1,000,000). We thus simulated 1,000,000 populations with 10,000 individuals in each population by creating data sets populated with 10,000 data points using SAS statistical software. We generated exposure probabilities for each of these populations. Each data point (individual in the population) had a preset probability of each exposure (genetic risk variant [G], environmental factor [E], and background rate [X]); we used a random number generator and a binomial probability distribution to assign individuals as exposed or unexposed. The exposures were assumed to be uncorrelated. The preset probability of individuals in each population having G ranged from 1% to 100% in each population; similar ranges were possible for E and X. We used 1,000,000 populations so the full range of the intersection of all probabilities could be exposed.

3.3 Analysis

We present in the results nine scenarios for the prevalence of environmental factors and the background prevalence of disease. These include prevalences of E and X likely to be found at the population level for most chronic disease (e.g., low background rate, moderate to high prevalence of environmental factors) as well as prevalences that are extreme (e.g., background rates of disease >80%). These thresholds were selected to be illustrative; the full results for any threshold are available on request. The nine scenarios are as follows:

1. Low prevalence of E (1%–5%), low prevalence of X (1%–5%)
2. Low prevalence of E (1%-5%), moderate prevalence of X (25%–35%)
3. Low prevalence of E (1%–5%), high prevalence of X (>80%)
4. Moderate prevalence of E (25%–35%), low prevalence of X (1%–5%)
5. Moderate prevalence of E (25%–35%), moderate prevalence of X (25%–35%)
6. Moderate prevalence of E (25%–35%), high prevalence of X (>80%)
7. High prevalence of E (>80%), low prevalence of X (1%–5%)
8. High prevalence of E (>80%), moderate prevalence of X (25%–35%)
9. High prevalence of E (>80%), high prevalence of X (>80%)

We estimated the risk of disease among those exposed to G compared with the risk of disease among those unexposed to G at every possible prevalence of G in the population from 1% to 100% with each of the nine scenarios. This risk ratio and risk difference was then estimated, using basic categorical data analysis in the SAS statistical software program. Statistical testing was unnecessary because these are simulated populations rather than samples.

3.4 Prediction When There Is Interaction: Results from the Simulation

Figure 10.1 shows nine separate graphs with G prevalence in each of 100 populations on the *x*-axis and risk ratio magnitude on the *y*-axis. In Figure 10.2, we show the same scenarios, with the measure of association being the risk difference rather than the risk ratio. Four results of note emerge from this series of simulations.

3.4.1 At Any G Prevalence, the Determinant of the Magnitude of the Risk Ratio and the Risk Difference Is Prevalence of E and X

Based on Figure 10.1, in six of nine graphs, the line for the magnitude of the risk ratio by gene prevalence (P) is almost perfectly flat. For example, when P(E) is high and P(X) is moderate, the risk ratio for the effect of G on the outcome is around 2.0, both when G prevalence is 1% and when G prevalence is 99%.

There is variation, however, in the magnitude of the risk ratios when we examine across different graphs. Examining the three graphs in the row where P(X) is moderate, we see the risk ratio associated with G, at any prevalence, is

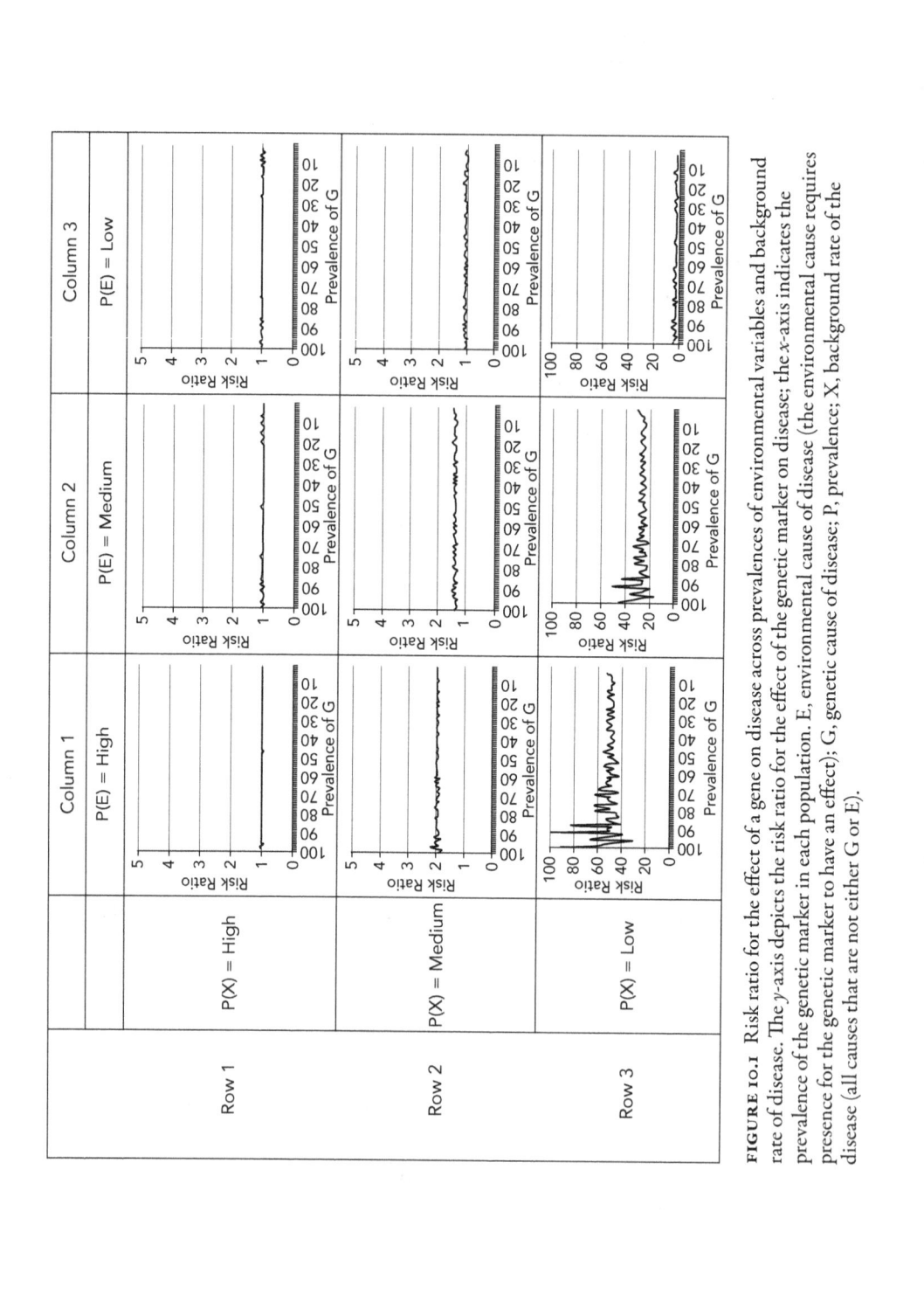

FIGURE 10.1 Risk ratio for the effect of a gene on disease across prevalences of environmental variables and background rate of disease. The y-axis depicts the risk ratio for the effect of the genetic marker on disease; the x-axis indicates the prevalence of the genetic marker in each population. E, environmental cause of disease (the environmental cause requires presence for the genetic marker to have an effect); G, genetic cause of disease; P, prevalence; X, background rate of the disease (all causes that are not either G or E).

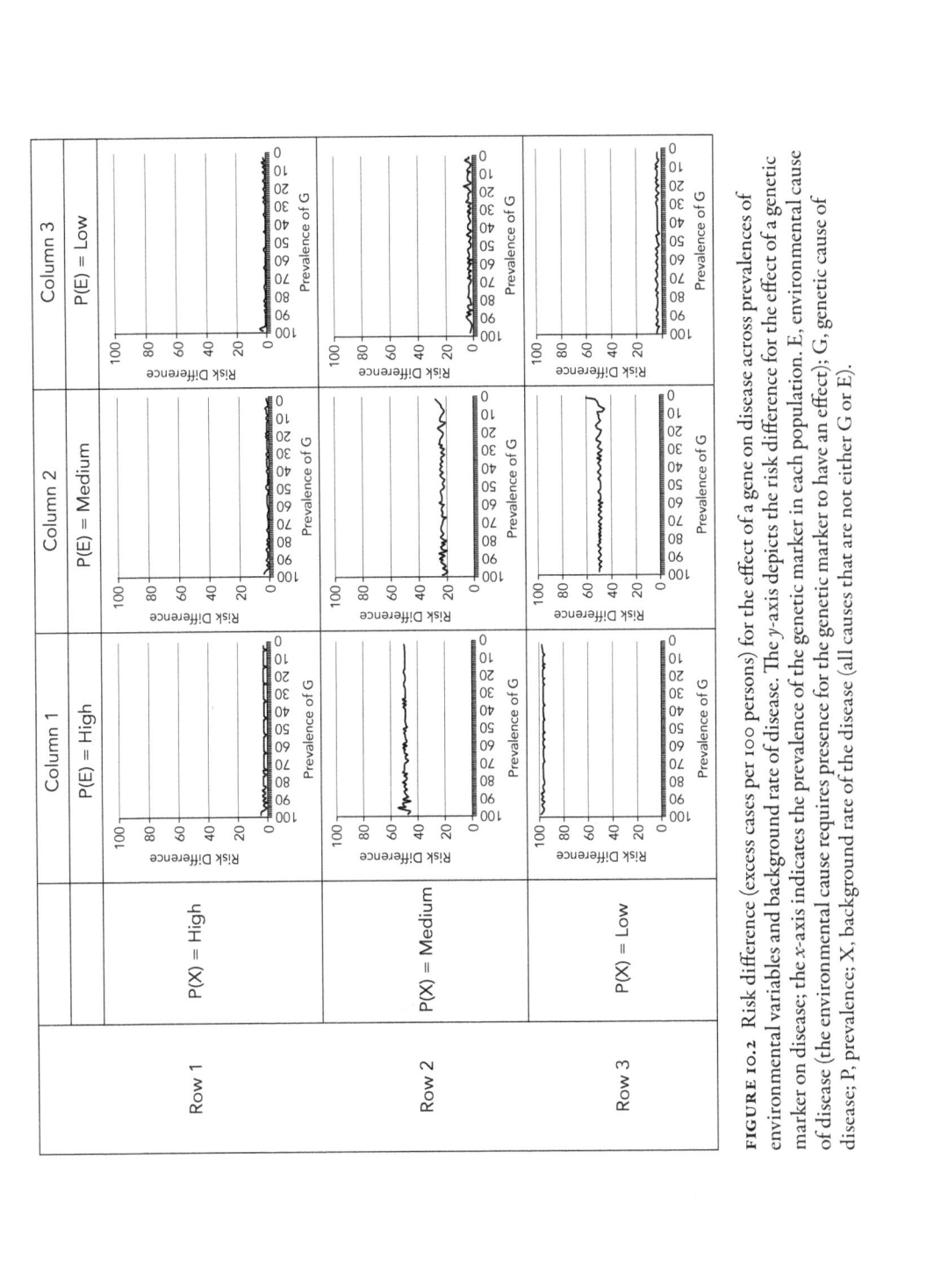

FIGURE 10.2 Risk difference (excess cases per 100 persons) for the effect of a gene on disease across prevalences of environmental variables and background rate of disease. The y-axis depicts the risk difference for the effect of a genetic marker on disease; the x-axis indicates the prevalence of the genetic marker in each population. E, environmental cause of disease (the environmental cause requires presence for the genetic marker to have an effect); G, genetic cause of disease; P, prevalence; X, background rate of the disease (all causes that are not either G or E).

around 2.0 when P(E) is high, is around 1.5 when P(E) is moderate, and is 1.0 when P(E) is low. Thus, the determinant of the size of the risk ratio associated with G is the prevalence of the environmental factors that activates it.

Similarly, based on Figure 10.2, the risk difference is constant at all prevalences of G when P(E) and P(X) are held constant, whether P(E) is high or low, or whether P(X) is high or low. The risk difference changes as P(E) and P(X) change, but not within particular P(E) and P(X) levels across prevalences of G.

3.4.2 At Every G Prevalence, the Risk Ratio and the Risk Difference Increases as the Prevalence of E Increases

When the prevalence of the background rate is less than 80% (as it will be in almost all conceivable circumstances), there is an increase in the risk ratio and the risk difference associated with G with increasing prevalence of E. This increase is, again, invariant to the prevalence of G. Thus, holding the background rate constant and less than 80%, if the prevalence of E increases, the magnitude of the association between G and the disease also increases. Note the prevalence of G does not vary the size of the risk ratio.

Similarly, the risk difference also increases with increasing prevalence of E. For example, when the background rate is moderate, the disease is attributable to an excess of five cases of disease per 100 persons when P(E) is almost ubiquitous, and almost no cases of disease when P(E) is very rare. When the environmental cause of disease is ubiquitous and the background rate of disease is low, virtually all cases of disease within the population are attributable to G.

3.4.3 At Every G Prevalence, the Risk Ratio Decreases as the Background Rate of Disease Increases

As shown in columns 1 and 2 of Figure 10.1, as long as the prevalence of E is greater than 5%, the risk ratio associated with G decreases as the background rate increases. The same pattern is found for risk differences (Figure 10.2). The excess cases of disease attributable to genetic variance decreases as the background rate of disease increases. That is, as more individuals in the population are exposed to factors that cause disease, regardless of whether they have the risk-raising genetic variant, the fewer the individuals in that population who will acquire the disease from the interaction of G and E.

3.4.4 When the Background Rate Is Low, There Is More Variability in the Effect of G on Disease When the Prevalence of G Is Low

We now turn our attention to the one scenario in which the prevalence of G matters for the magnitude of the association between G and the disease.

Examining the third row of Figure 10.1, we see there is variability in the magnitude of the risk ratio associated with G when the prevalence of the genetic variant is low in the population and the prevalence of E is greater than 5%. However, the risk ratio associated with the genetic variant in these scenarios is large regardless. In the first column, the risk ratio ranges from 38.0 to 100.0; in the second column, the risk ratio ranges from 20.0 to 40.0. In the third column, the modal risk ratio is 3.0 but ranges from 1 to 5.

Risk differences, in contrast, are more stable across the range of gene prevalences when the background rate is low, likely as a result of the inherent bounds of an additive measure to be between 0 and 100 compared with a multiplicative measure such as the risk ratio, which can take on values from zero to infinity.

4.0 Summary: Prediction of Disease in the Presence of Interaction

Using simulations that span the range of potential possible prevalences of genes, environmental factors, and unrelated factors, we show the magnitude of both the risk ratio and the risk difference association between a genetic factor and health outcome depends entirely on the prevalence of two factors: (1) the factors that interact with the genetic variant of interest and (2) the background rate of disease in the population. These results indicate that genetic risk factors can predict disease adequately only in the presence of common interacting factors, suggesting natural limits on the predictive ability of individual risk factors to predict disease based on co-occurring factors with the individual risk factor.

Genetic epidemiological investigations have, for some chronic diseases, moved toward multilocus gene scores rather than single variants, with the goal of improving predictability. However, the concepts we illustrate here can be translated to any germline genetic variant or score. The ability of these multilocus scores to predict disease occurrence depends entirely on the prevalence of the environmental factors that interact with the genetic factors in the multilocus score. Furthermore, if there is heterogeneity in the interaction of environmental factors with the variety of genetic factors across the score, the predictability of the multilocus gene score may vary substantially across populations. This is perfectly in line with the concepts we introduced at the beginning of the chapter regarding positive predictive value; predictive value increases as prevalence of the various factors that interact disease also increase.

More broadly, our simulation provides a guide for assessment of prediction. Fundamentally, risk factors for disease at a population level may have little predictive validity at the individual level. The predictive validity increases as the prevalence of the disease increases, the prevalence of factors that interact with the exposure of interest increases, and the prevalence of factors that also cause the disease but do not interact with the exposure of interest decreases. Yet, we are working with averages in population health and factors that may be broadly distal to the mechanism through which the disease occurs.

This underlies our ninth principle of population health science (Box 10.1). That is, given information about the population distributions of health and disease, we identify factors that predict the averages within and across populations, yet these averages may not identify which individuals in those populations will develop the illness. Despite our inability to give individuals an accurate probability of whether they will get sick, population averages are incredibly useful tools for public health. Our public health recommendations and programs are often based on what is optimal for the population rather than for individuals, including smoke-free air, vaccination, healthy food options, and policies that promote equality in treatment and access to safe housing. None of these will likely benefit all or even the majority of individuals, and in fact there may be risks as well as tradeoffs for the individual. For example, there are rare but present adverse effects of vaccination, yet the benefits to the community of high levels of vaccination are clear. Furthermore, if we could predict with accuracy who would develop heart disease from a high-fat diet, then some could enjoy all the onion rings they could muster if they knew they were at very low risk. Because we cannot predict such events with accuracy, we promote healthy diets for all. Such are the complexities of population health science. Efforts to establish prediction in population health will undoubtedly continue and—with careful and rigorous measurement of risk factors and their interactions—may be beneficial. We should always, however, keep in mind our population health principles considering averages, the good for the population, and differences across populations that are meaningful for continued assessment of health across systems and levels.

BOX 10.1

Ninth Foundational Principle of Population Health Science

We can predict health in populations with much more certainty than we can predict health in individuals.

5.0 References

Bayer, R., and S. Galea. (2015). Public health in the precision-medicine era. *N Engl J Med* **373**(6): 499–501.

Bellcross, C. A., P. Z. Page, and D. Meaney-Delman. (2012). Direct-to-consumer personal genome testing and cancer risk prediction. *Cancer J* **18**(4): 293–302.

Collins, F. S., and V. A. McKusick. (2001). Implications of the Human Genome Project for medical science. *JAMA* **285**(5): 540–544.

Collins, F. S., and H. Varmus. (2015). A new initiative on precision medicine. *N Engl J Med* **372**(9): 793–795.

D'Agostino, R. B., Sr., S. Grundy, L. M. Sullivan, P. Wilson, and CHD Risk Prediction Group. (2001). Validation of the Framingham coronary heart disease prediction scores: results of a multiple ethnic group investigation. *JAMA* **286**(2): 180–187.

Davey Smith, G. (2011). Use of genetic markers and gene–diet interactions for interrogating population-level causal influences of diet on health. *Genes Nutr* **6**(1): 27–43.

Eisenberg, A. (2013). Genomic analysis: the Office Edition. *New York Times*.

Hamburg, M. A., and F. S. Collins. (2010). The path to personalized medicine. *N Engl J Med* **363**(4): 301–304.

Hood, L., and M. Flores. (2012). A personal view on systems medicine and the emergence of proactive P4 medicine: predictive, preventive, personalized and participatory. *N Biotechnol* **29**(6): 613–624.

Janssens, A. C., and C. M. van Duijn. (2008). Genome-based prediction of common diseases: advances and prospects. *Hum Mol Genet* **17**(R2): R166–R173.

Khoury, M. J., M. L. Gwinn, R. E. Glasgow, and B. S. Kramer. (2012). A population approach to precision medicine. *Am J Prev Med* **42**(6): 639–645.

Kirkman, M. A., P. Yu-Wai-Man, A. Korsten, M. Leonhardt, K. Dimitriadis, I. F. De Coo, et al. (2009). Gene–environment interactions in Leber hereditary optic neuropathy. *Brain* **132**(Pt 9): 2317–2326.

Lawlor, D. A., G. D. Smith, and S. Ebrahim. (2004). Association between childhood socioeconomic status and coronary heart disease risk among postmenopausal women: findings from the British Women's Heart and Health Study. *Am J Public Health* **94**(8): 1386–1392.

Luo, H., I. Burstyn, and P. Gustafson. (2013). Investigations of gene–disease associations: costs and benefits of environmental data. *Epidemiology* **24**(4): 562–568.

Major Depressive Disorder Working Group of the Psychiatric Genome-Wide Association Studies (GWAS) Consortium, S. Ripke, N. R. Wray, C. M. Lewis, S. P. Hamilton, M. M. Weissman, et al. (2013). A mega-analysis of genome-wide association studies for major depressive disorder. *Mol Psychiatry* **18**(4): 497–511.

Manolio, T. A., F. S. Collins, N. J. Cox, D. B. Goldstein, L. A. Hindorff, D. J. Hunter, et al. (2009). Finding the missing heritability of complex diseases. *Nature* **461**(7265): 747–753.

Ong, F. S., K. Das, J. Wang, H. Vakil, J. Z. Kuo, W. L. Blackwell, et al. (2012). Personalized medicine and pharmacogenetic biomarkers: progress in molecular oncology testing. *Expert Rev Mol Diagn* **12**(6): 593–602.

Pepe, M. S., H. Janes, G. Longton, W. Leisenring, and P. Newcomb. (2004). Limitations of the odds ratio in gauging the performance of a diagnostic, prognostic, or screening marker. *Am J Epidemiol* **159**(9): 882–890.

Prainsack, B., J. Reardon, R. Hindmarsh, H. Gottweis, U. Naue, and J. E. Lunshof. (2008). Personal genomes: misdirected precaution. *Nature* **456**(7218): 34–35.

Rothman, K., S. Greenland, and T. L. Lash. (2008). *Modern epidemiology* (3rd edition). Philadelphia, PA: Lippincott, Williams & Wilkins.

Smith, G. D. (2011). Epidemiology, epigenetics and the 'gloomy prospect': embracing randomness in population health research and practice. *Int J Epidemiol* **40**(3): 537–562.

Smith, G. D., C. Hart, D. Blane, and D. Hole. (1998). Adverse socioeconomic conditions in childhood and cause specific adult mortality: prospective observational study. *BMJ* **316**(7145): 1631–1635.

Voight, B. F., G. M. Peloso, M. Orho-Melander, R. Frikke-Schmidt, M. Barbalic, M. K. Jensen, et al. (2012). Plasma HDL cholesterol and risk of myocardial infarction: a Mendelian randomisation study. *Lancet* **380**(9841): 572–580.

Wilson, P. W., R. B. D'Agostino, D. Levy, A. M. Belanger, H. Silbershatz, and W. B. Kannel. (1998). Prediction of coronary heart disease using risk factor categories. *Circulation* **97**(18): 1837–1847.

Wolf, P. A., R. B. D'Agostino, A. J. Belanger, and W. B. Kannel. (1991). Probability of stroke: a risk profile from the Framingham Study. *Stroke* **22**(3): 312–318.

Wray, N. R., J. Yang, B. J. Hayes, A. L. Price, M. E. Goddard, and P. M. Visscher. (2013). Pitfalls of predicting complex traits from SNPs. *Nat Rev Genet* **14**(7): 507–515.

Wright, C. F., and S. Gregory-Jones. (2010). Size of the direct-to-consumer genomic testing market. *Genet Med* **12**(9): 594.

11

Case Study

CAN WE REDUCE OBESITY BY ENCOURAGING
PEOPLE TO EAT HEALTHY FOOD?

Jonathan Platt, Katherine M. Keyes, and Sandro Galea

IN THIS CHAPTER and in Chapter 12 we present two case studies, both about topics of immediate relevance and salience to population health scientists. It is our goal in these chapters to illustrate how the principles we develop throughout this book inform our thinking about particular health indicators and how we might approach prevention efforts.

In the United States, an estimated 17% of children age 2 to 19 years are considered obese and 32% are overweight (Ogden et al. 2014). Worldwide, between 12.9% and 23.8% of children are obese, and the prevalence is increasing (Ng et al. 2014). Preventing the onset of obesity remains a critical public health goal for the next decade (Olshansky et al. 2005). Such primary prevention efforts require an investment in childhood, given that 12.9% of children are already obese by age 5 years, and the risk of obesity by eighth grade is four times greater in overweight versus normal-weight 5-year-olds (Cunningham et al. 2014). Furthermore, overweight children are at least twice as likely to become overweight adults than normal-weight children. This risk is even greater among obese children (Whitaker et al. 1997, Singh et al. 2008).

The United States is substantially invested in efforts to tackle this challenge. In particular, investment has aimed at encouraging change in individual and family behavior toward food and exercise. For example, the American Academy of Pediatrics guidelines to reduce obesity in children and adolescents focus on personalized weight, diet, and physical activity management strategies (Gidding et al. 2006, U.S. Department of Health and Human

Services 2008). These guidelines underpin two primary goals of the high-profile White House initiative led by First Lady Michelle Obama, called *Let's Move*. First, a child's BMI should be calculated during routine clinical visits and be given to parents with guidance on how to achieve a healthy weight. Second, guidelines and information about the impact of healthy eating habits and regular physical activity should be given to families during clinical visits.

These approaches, however, assume that a focus on changing individual and family behavior, and on the importance of in-person clinician visits for obesity consultation, will be effective in reducing the population burden of obesity onset. But will it? Certainly, eating less and exercising more are time-tested approaches to weight management. Yet, there is often a wide chasm between what we know will produce good results (eat well, exercise regularly) and how we go about producing those results (Horodyska et al. 2015). Empirically, it remains unclear whether, at a population level, interventions that encourage individual-level behavior change will have a meaningful impact on population rates of childhood obesity. For example, the effects of an intervention that promotes healthy eating and physical activity may be different across families with varying prevalences of other risk factors for obesity and those in neighborhoods characterized by different walkability and safety (Papas et al. 2007, Sekhobo et al. 2014). Therefore, although individuals who do eat well and exercise more will lose weight, this does not necessarily mean wholesale efforts to encourage better individual behavior will result in obesity changing in entire populations.

Any discussion of how to intervene on obesity needs to rest on an understanding of the causes of obesity, the prevalence of these causes, and how amenable these causes are to intervention. Fortunately, in the case of obesity, the causes are well studied, and the literature reflects a broad range of factors including—interindividual variation in genetic susceptibility and metabolism (Frayling et al. 2004, Friedman 2004, O'Rahilly and Farooqi 2008), personality (Gerlach et al. 2015), family influences such as food preferences and sedentary lifestyle (Soubhi et al. 2004, Gruber and Haldeman 2009), individual decisions about consumption and activity (Hill and Peters 1998), built environmental characteristics (Papas et al. 2007), food prices (Drewnowski 2004), access to green space (Bedimo-Rung et al. 2005, Liu et al. 2007, Bell et al. 2008), and safe neighborhoods (Lovasi et al. 2013).

This large number of causes then suggests there are many potential routes toward intervention. Thus, although *Let's Move* and other similar campaigns have placed stock in motivating individual behavior change, choosing this approach necessitates shifting focus from other approaches. In a world of finite resources, this is very much a choice to invest in one area but not others. But, is this the right place for us to invest if we want to reduce obesity?

1.0 Causal Structure of Obesity

The principles of population health science offer much to help guide us in addressing the question of the right place or places to invest to reduce obesity. Here we illustrate how to conceptualize the limits of individual-level behavioral interventions on the population distributions of obesity incidence using basic assumptions and data simulation. We begin our simulation by creating a causal structure for obesity operating on three levels: macrosocial, individual, and molecular. The macrosocial environment includes all factors related to availability of food, food policy, built environment, and accessibility of safe areas for physical activity (termed *unhealthy environment* moving forward). The individual level includes family and individual approaches to weight control (e.g., promoting physical activity and healthy eating), called *individual motivation*. The molecular level includes genetic vulnerability to obesity through both common germline mutations and gene disorders. It is inarguable that macrosocial, individual, and molecular factors all matter to the production of obesity. Building on the available literature, we specify here that an unhealthy environment interacts with individual motivation in causing obesity, such that individual motivation only has an effect on preventing obesity when not in an unhealthy environment. Furthermore, we specify that genetic vulnerability to obesity sets a general background rate of obesity independent of unhealthy environments and individual motivations. Table 11.1 summarizes the causal architecture we specify in this chapter. Those who become obese are those who are exposed to both an unhealthy environment and individual determinants, or those who are exposed to genetic risk.

These assumptions are made while readily acknowledging simplifications. We are not accounting for the social networks and interactions among the macrosocial, individual, and molecular determinants that constitute a complex ecosystem (Auchincloss et al. 2011, El-Sayed et al. 2013). Furthermore, we are focusing on just two factors in a complex set that influence obesity. However, our simulation extends the typical approach to the development of obesity that focuses on only one causal level. Our approach is intended to abstract such an ecosystem and focus on one particular element—interaction across levels, which undoubtedly exists—within the system.

In this simulation there is a baseline proportion of individuals who will become obese regardless of the food environment or their individual

160   POPULATION HEALTH SCIENCE

Table 11.1 Causal Architecture of Obesity for Simulation

Exposed to Individual Determinants, I	Exposed to Unhealthy Environment, E	Genetically Vulnerable, X	Presence of Obesity
0	0	0	No
0	0	1	Yes
0	1	0	No
0	1	1	Yes
1	1	1	Yes
1	0	0	No
1	0	1	Yes
1	1	0	Yes

0, unexposed; 1, exposed. Individuals in the simulated populations become obese if exposed to both individual determinants and an unhealthy environment, or if they are genetically vulnerable.

motivation (we henceforth term these individuals *genetically vulnerable*); we vary that baseline proportion as part of the simulation. Among the remainder of individuals, obesity will occur through a combination of unhealthy environment and individual motivation (i.e., individuals become obese when exposed to both an unhealthy environment and when lacking individual motivation to engage with physical activity and healthy diet); we vary the proportion exposed to an unhealthy environment and the proportion exposed to individual motivation throughout the simulation as well. The proportions that are genetically vulnerable are called X; unhealthy environment, E; and individual motivation, I.

2.0   Simulated Populations

For this simulation we used the same basis as the simulation presented in Chapter 10. We simulate 1,000,000 populations with 10,000 individuals in each population. We then generated exposure probabilities for each of these populations. Each individual in the population has a preset probability of each exposure (genetic vulnerability [X], unhealthy environment [E], and individual motivation [I]); we used a random number generator and a binomial probability distribution to assign individuals as exposed or unexposed to each of the three exposures. The exposures are assumed to be uncorrelated with each other. The preset probability of individuals in each population having E ranges from 1% to 100% in each population; similar ranges are possible for

I and the X. We use 1,000,000 populations so the full range of the intersection of all probabilities is exposed. For example, in 100 populations, the probability of E (i.e., proportion exposed to an unhealthy environment) is 1% and the probability of X (i.e., proportion genetically vulnerable) is 1%; the probability of I ranges from 1% to 100% across these populations. In another 100 populations, the probability of E is 2% and X is 1%; the probability of I ranges from 1% to 100% across these 100 populations. We vary all possible combinations of the three parameters, thus generating 1,000,000 populations.

3.0 Analysis

We estimate the risk of obesity among those lacking individual motivation (P[Y]|I = 1) compared with the risk of obesity among those not lacking individual motivation (P[Y]|I = 0), where Y is a binary indicator of obesity (BMI, >95th percentile). The proportion of population with individual motivation (I) varies in each population.

From these risk estimates, we derive two summaries. First, we derive the total number of cases of obesity in the population, out of each population of 10,000. This is estimated by summing the number of cases among those exposed with the number of cases among those unexposed. Second, we estimate the population attributable risk proportion (PARP) resulting from having individual motivation as

$$(P([Y]|I = 1) - \frac{P([Y]|I = 0)}{P([Y]|I = 1)},$$

representing the excess cases caused by change in individual motivation.

We present the analytic results in two ways. First, we present results for just two of the million populations we simulated to show the contrasting results that can be obtained when changing the population prevalence of unhealthy environment. Based on existing literature, we estimate that 75% of children can be categorized as regularly engaging in physical activity; thus, we set the prevalence of individual motivation as 75% in both populations (Veerman 2011, Fakhouri et al. 2014, Qi et al. 2014). Also based on empirical literature, we set the prevalence of genetic vulnerability at 5% in both populations (Veerman 2011, Fakhouri et al. 2014, Qi et al. 2014). The only factor that varies across the two populations is unhealthy environment. In population A, only 1% of children are exposed to an unhealthy environment. In population B, 80% of children are exposed to an unhealthy environment.

Second, we expand to present the results for 900 of the 1,000,000 populations analyzed, which is sufficient to demonstrate the central theses of the findings. We construct nine scenarios, with 100 populations in each scenario, in which the prevalence of the unhealthy environment and the prevalence of genetic vulnerability is set within each scenario whereas the prevalence of individual motivation differs.

Within each scenario, we present the number of obesity cases and the PARP for 100 populations, with the prevalence of unhealthy choices ranging from 1% to 100%. We then graph two parameters for every population: (1) the total number of cases of obesity and (2) the PARP resulting from unhealthy choices.

4.0 Results

4.1 Results from Two Populations: Same Level of Individual Motivation, Same Prevalence of Genetic Vulnerability, Different Prevalence of Unhealthy Environment

Across the two populations, individual motivations only have an effect in the context of a prevalent unhealthy environment. The results indicate that in population A there is no association between individual determinants and obesity risk, with a risk ratio of 1.01, risk difference of zero, and a PARP of 0.005, which indicates that almost no obesity in the population is attributable to individual determinants of obesity. In population B, in contrast, those exposed to individual determinants of obesity have approximately 15.2 times the risk of developing obesity compared with those unexposed to individual determinants, and almost all 93% of the obesity in the population is attributable to individual determinants. Because individual determinants interact with the broader environment in our simulation, the results indicate that individual determinants explain obesity patterns only when the prevalence of the factor with which they interact (in our simulation, the healthiness of the broader environment) is high.

4.2 Results from 900 Populations: For Three Levels of Unhealthy Environment and Genetic Vulnerability, Different Level of Individual Motivation

Figure 11.1 shows nine separate graphs with I prevalence (the proportion exposed to individual determinants) in each of 100 populations on the x-axis and number of individuals with obesity on the y-axis. In Figure 11.2, we show

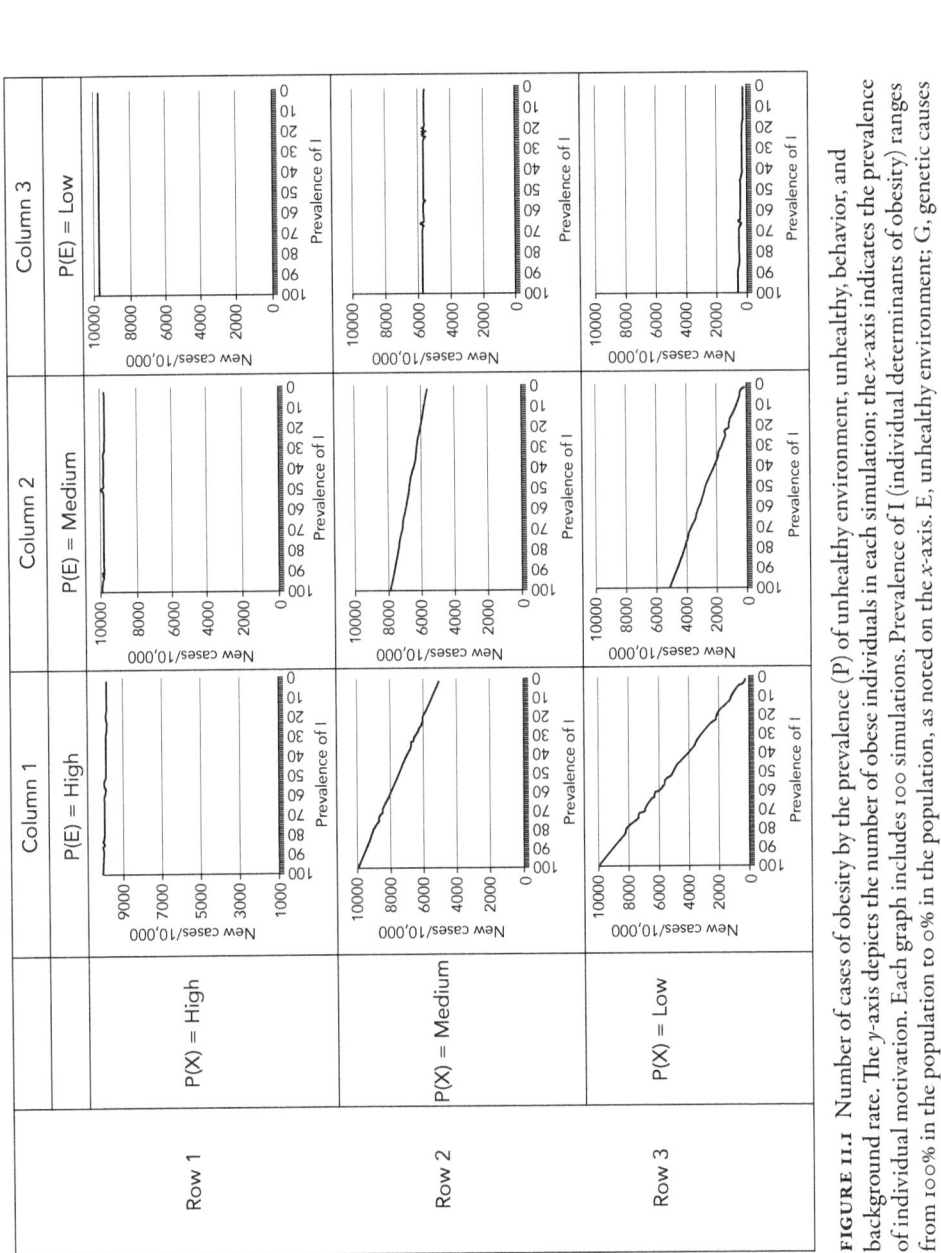

FIGURE 11.1 Number of cases of obesity by the prevalence (P) of unhealthy environment, unhealthy, behavior, and background rate. The y-axis depicts the number of obese individuals in each simulation; the x-axis indicates the prevalence of individual motivation. Each graph includes 100 simulations. Prevalence of I (individual determinants of obesity) ranges from 100% in the population to 0% in the population, as noted on the x-axis. E, unhealthy environment; G, genetic causes of obesity; I, individual motivation.

FIGURE 11.2 Population attributable risk proportion (PARP) for the effect of changing unhealthy behavior on obesity by the prevalence of unhealthy environment, prevalence of unhealthy behavior, and background rate. The y-axis depicts the PARP for the association between individual motivation and obesity; the x-axis indicates the prevalence of individual motivation. Each graph includes 100 simulations. Prevalence of I (individual determinants of obesity) ranges from 100% in the population to 0% in the population, as noted on the x-axis. E, unhealthy environment; G, genetic causes of obesity; I, individual motivation.

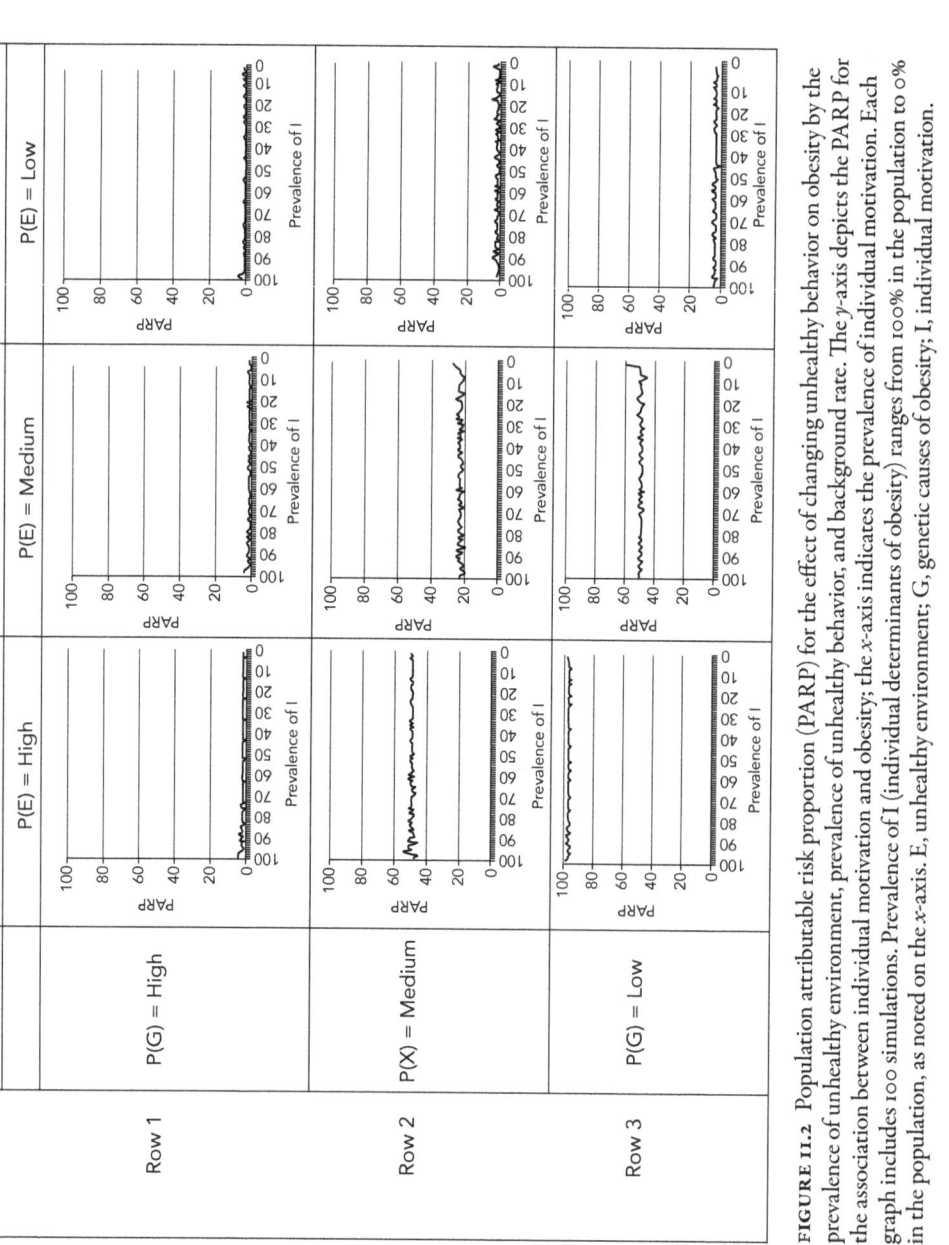

the same scenarios, with the PARP on the *y*-axis. Three results of note emerge from this series of simulations.

4.2.1 Individual Determinants Have No Impact on the Number of Obese Individuals in the Population When Few Are Exposed to an Unhealthy Environment

In column 3 of Figure 11.1, we see the number of obese individuals in each population under the restriction that exposure to unhealthy environments is low. In this scenario, the number of obese individuals is relatively constant regardless of the proportion of individuals who are exposed to individual determinants. For example, examining the graph in row 2, column 3 (exposure to unhealthy environments is low [1%–5%], when genetic vulnerability is moderate [25%–25%]), approximately 6000 individuals of 10,000 will be obese in a population when close to 100% of individuals make unhealthy choices. When the proportion of individuals who make unhealthy choices is close to 0%, the number of obese individuals is 5900. Examining the graphs across rows 1, 2, and 3 of column 3, we see the number of obese individuals; the slope of the line that determines the number of obese individuals across population prevalences of individual determinants is determined by the proportion who are genetically vulnerable to obesity, rather than individual determinants. This is because, in our scenario, individuals need to be exposed to both individual determinants of obesity and be in an unhealthy environment to become obese. When the environment is healthy (e.g., population prevalence exposed to unhealthy environment is low [between 1% and 5%]), no individuals will become obese, regardless of their exposure to individual determinants.

4.2.2 The Prevalence of Individual Determinants of Obesity Is Related to the Number of Cases of Obesity Only When the Unhealthy Environment Has Moderate to High Prevalence and When the Prevalence of Genetic Risk for Obesity Is Low

Examining the four scenarios in columns 1 and 2, in which the prevalence of exposure to an unhealthy environment is medium to high, we see a decline in the number of obese individuals in each population as the proportion of individuals who are exposed to individual determinants decreases. The steepest decline is seen in column 1, row 3, when exposure to an unhealthy environment is ubiquitous and the proportion exposed to genetic vulnerability is low. In this scenario, each decrease in the proportion of individuals who make unhealthy choices translates to a decrease in approximately 100 cases of obesity per 10,000 individuals.

4.2.3 The PARP for the Association Between Individual Determinants and Obesity Does Not Vary Across the Prevalence of Individual Choice When the Proportion Exposed to Unhealthy Environments and the Prevalence of Genetic Risk Factors Is Constant

Shown in Figure 11.2 is the proportion of obesity attributable to individual determinants in each of the nine scenarios. Within each scenario, there is little variability of the PARP based on the prevalence of individuals exposed to individual determinants. For example, when the prevalence of individuals exposed to an unhealthy environment is ubiquitous and the proportion exposed to genetic vulnerability is low (column 1, row 3), all cases of obesity are attributable to individual determinant, regardless of the proportion of individuals who are exposed to individual determinants. The same is true when exposure to unhealthy environments is moderate (column 2, row 3). When exposure to unhealthy environments is low but genetic vulnerability is moderate or high, no cases are attributable to individual determinants, regardless of the proportion of people in the population who are exposed to individual determinants.

One way in which to conceptualize these simulations is as follows: when everyone is exposed to an unhealthy environment and few people will develop obesity because of genetic risk factors, the only reason one person becomes obese and another does not is because of exposure to individual determinants. When everyone is exposed to a healthy environment, conversely, exposure to individual determinants explains almost no cases of obesity, because the prevalence of exposure to unhealthy environments is so rare.

5.0 A Population Health Science Approach to Obesity Prevention: Conclusions

Alarmed by the obesity epidemic, a global effort is underway to ask individuals to reduce their risk of obesity by eating healthy food and exercising more. Will such an approach work to reduce the population burden of obesity? We have addressed this question through a series of simple assumptions about the causal architecture of obesity, recognizing that individual approaches to weight management vary in their effect across broader environmental contexts that promote or hinder individual choices. This approach finds the effect of individual motivations to prevent obesity, such as encouraging children and their families to eat healthy food and exercise more, is bounded by the prevalence of the unhealthy environment in which the children are living. This prevalence greatly affects both the number of incident obesity cases we observe and the proportion attributable to individual determinants.

In some respects, these results might seem perplexing. Surely if everyone ate healthier and exercised more, obesity would decrease in populations, yes? However, we know there is a less than perfect correlation between attempting to motivate individuals to engage in positive health behaviors and the health behaviors themselves. In fact, there is good evidence the link is quite weak between telling individuals to do something and then subsequently seeing demonstrable shifts in long-term behavior (Ussher et al. 2014, Horodyska et al. 2015). Therefore, the operative issue is not whether everyone eating less and exercising more would reduce the population prevalence of obesity. The solution to this issue, clearly, is yes. Rather, the operative question is: What should we do to improve obesity in populations? We submit that the answer to this question may have little to do with telling people how to behave.

What matters more—individual motivation to change behavior or unhealthy environments—depends on the assumptions we make about the casual architecture of their co-occurrence as well as prevalence in the population. However, at its core, the central assumption that underlies this analysis is that both individual behaviors and environments matter to produce obesity in populations. This is demonstrated abundantly in the literature (Vandenbroeck et al. 2007). Motivating individual behavior change can only be effective under the explicit condition that the factors that interact with behavior change are ubiquitously present in the population. More broadly, the potential to reduce the population burden of obesity by focusing on promoting individual-level approaches to changes in health behavior can be conceptualized only in the context of the prevalence of unhealthy environments.

Although, conceptually, it may seem obvious that by changing the broader environment while simultaneously changing individual motivation we can have maximal impact on the population prevalence of obesity, this is a premise not fully appreciated in much of the literature or in public comments and actions on obesity. We demonstrate here the mathematical reality that, although still a cause of obesity, individual motivation to prevent the onset of obesity has no impact on the population prevalence even when 100% of the population is motivated individually under certain conditions of the broader social environment (e.g. lack of access to nutritious foods, lack of space to exercise).

The principles demonstrated in this simulation are fundamental to quantitative population health science. Population health science as a discipline rests on the notion that the drivers that shift health are often not only ubiquitous and unseen, but also etiologically and conceptually distinct, and linked to those factors that differentiate the healthy from the sick within populations (Rose 1985). Furthermore, those indicators we consider to have relatively strong associations with health indicators within populations actually do a poor job of predicting who will become sick at an individual level (Pepe et al. 2004, Keyes et al. 2015). And finally, ample evidence indicates the factors we consider to have strong associations within a population, across a wide range of health indicators, change demonstrably across populations (Rothman et al. 2008, Poole 2010).

The limitations of our approach center around the utility of the model we estimate for our simulation. We specified there was an interaction between an unhealthy environment and individual motivations, such that, for some children, both were necessary to become obese. We also specified there was another pathway to becoming obese: being genetically vulnerable. The evidence that identified genetic risk factors for obesity may potentially interact with both the built environment and with individual action such as physical activity is mixed, with evidence both for and against (Andreasen et al. 2008, Corella et al. 2012, Foraita et al. 2015). However, our principal argument is that individual motivation is bounded in effects by the prevalence of factors that interact with them. Thus, if genetic factors interact with individual motivation, then again the effects of individual motivation on population rates of obesity will be bounded by the prevalence of the risk alleles for development of obesity. Furthermore, we note the actual process of caloric intake and physical activity are ultimately mediators of all the effects we specify here.

6.0 References

Andreasen, C. H., K. L. Stender-Petersen, M. S. Mogensen, S. S. Torekov, L. Wegner, G. Andersen, et al. (2008). Low physical activity accentuates the effect of the FTO rs9939609 polymorphism on body fat accumulation. *Diabetes* **57**(1): 95–101.

Auchincloss, A. H., R. L. Riolo, D. G. Brown, J. Cook, and A. V. Diez Roux. (2011). An agent-based model of income inequalities in diet in the context of residential segregation. *Am J Prev Med* **40**(3): 303–311.

Bedimo-Rung, A. L., A. J. Mowen, and D. A. Cohen. (2005). The significance of parks to physical activity and public health: a conceptual model. *Am J Prev Med* **28**(2 Suppl 2): 159–168.

Bell, J. F., J. S. Wilson, and G. C. Liu. (2008). Neighborhood greenness and 2-year changes in body mass index of children and youth. *Am J Prev Med* **35**(6): 547–553.

Corella, D., P. Carrasco, J. V. Sorli, O. Coltell, C. Ortega-Azorin, M. Guillen, et al. (2012). Education modulates the association of the FTO rs9939609 polymorphism with body mass index and obesity risk in the Mediterranean population. *Nutr Metab Cardiovasc Dis* **22**(8): 651–658.

Cunningham, S. A., M. R. Kramer, and K. M. Narayan. (2014). Incidence of childhood obesity in the United States. *N Engl J Med* **370**(5): 403–411.

Drewnowski, A. (2004). Obesity and the food environment: dietary energy density and diet costs. *Am J Prev Med* **27**(3 Suppl): 154–162.

El-Sayed, A. M., L. Seemann, P. Scarborough, and S. Galea. (2013). Are network-based interventions a useful antiobesity strategy? An application of simulation models for causal inference in epidemiology. *Am J Epidemiol* **178**(2): 287–295.

Fakhouri, T. H., J. P. Hughes, V. L. Burt, M. Song, J. E. Fulton, and C. L. Ogden. (2014). Physical activity in U.S. youth aged 12—15 years, 2012. *NCHS Data Brief* **141**: 1–8.

Foraita, R., F. Gunther, W. Gwozdz, L. A. Reisch, P. Russo, F. Lauria, et al. (2015). Does the FTO gene interact with the socioeconomic status on the obesity development among young European children? Results from the IDEFICS study. *Int J Obes (Lond)* **39**(1): 1–6.

Frayling, T. M., N. J. Timpson, M. N. Weedon, E. Zeggini, R. M. Freathy, C. M. Lindgren, et al. (2004). Modern science versus the stigma of obesity. *Nat Med* **10**(6): 563–569.

Friedman, J. M. (2004). Modern science versus the stigma of obesity. *Nat Med* **10**(6): 563–569.

Gerlach, G., S. Herpertz, and S. Loeber. (2015). Personality traits and obesity: a systematic review. *Obes Rev* **16**(1): 32–63.

Gidding, S. S., B. A. Dennison, L. L. Birch, S. R. Daniels, M. W. Gillman, A. H. Lichtenstein, et al. (2006). Dietary recommendations for children and adolescents: a guide for practitioners. *Pediatrics* **117**(2): 544–559.

Gruber, K. J., and L. A. Haldeman. (2009). Using the family to combat childhood and adult obesity. *Prev Chronic Dis* **6**(3): A106.

Hill, J. O., and J. C. Peters. (1998). Environmental contributions to the obesity epidemic. *Science* **280**(5368): 1371–1374.

Horodyska, K., A. Luszczynska, M. van den Berg, M. Hendriksen, G. Roos, I. De Bourdeaudhuij, et al. (2015). Good practice characteristics of diet and physical activity interventions and policies: an umbrella review. *BMC Public Health* **15**: 19.

Keyes, K. M., G. D. Smith, K. C. Koenen, and S. Galea. (2015). The mathematical limits of genetic prediction for complex chronic disease. *J Epidemiol Commun Health* **69**(6): 574–579.

Liu, G. C., J. S. Wilson, R. Qi, and J. Ying. (2007). Green neighborhoods, food retail and childhood overweight: differences by population density. *Am J Health Promot* **21**(4 Suppl): 317–325.

Lovasi, G. S., O. Schwartz-Soicher, J. W. Quinn, D. K. Berger, K. M. Neckerman, R. Jaslow, et al. (2013). Neighborhood safety and green space as predictors of obesity among preschool children from low-income families in New York City. *Prev Med* **57**(3): 189–193.

Ng, M., T. Fleming, M. Robinson, B. Thomson, N. Graetz, C. Margono, et al. (2014). Global, regional, and national prevalence of overweight and obesity in children and adults during 1980–2013: a systematic analysis for the Global Burden of Disease Study 2013. *Lancet* **384**(9945): 766–781.

Ogden, C. L., M. D. Carroll, B. K. Kit, and K. M. Flegal. (2014). Prevalence of childhood and adult obesity in the United States, 2011–2012. *JAMA* **311**(8): 806–814.

Olshansky, S. J., D. J. Passaro, R. C. Hershow, J. Layden, B. A. Carnes, J. Brody, et al. (2005). A potential decline in life expectancy in the United States in the 21st century. *N Engl J Med* **352**(11): 1138–1145.

O'Rahilly, S., and I. S. Farooqi. (2008). Human obesity: a heritable neurobehavioral disorder that is highly sensitive to environmental conditions. *Diabetes* **57**(11): 2905–2910.

Papas, M. A., A. J. Alberg, R. Ewing, K. J. Helzlsouer, T. L. Gary, and A. C. Klassen. (2007). The built environment and obesity. *Epidemiol Rev* **29**: 129–143.

Pepe, M. S., H. Janes, G. Longton, W. Leisenring, and P. Newcomb. (2004). Limitations of the odds ratio in gauging the performance of a diagnostic, prognostic, or screening marker. *Am J Epidemiol* **159**(9): 882–890.

Poole, C. (2010). On the origin of risk relativism. *Epidemiology* **21**(1): 3–9.

Qi, Q., A. Y. Chu, J. H. Kang, J. Huang, L. M. Rose, M. K. Jensen, et al. (2014). Fried food consumption, genetic risk, and body mass index: gene–diet interaction analysis in three US cohort studies. *BMJ* **348**: g1610.

Rose, G. (1985). Sick individuals and sick populations. *Int J Epidemiol* **14**(1): 32–38.

Rothman, K., S. Greenland, and T. L. Lash. (2008). *Modern epidemiology* (3rd edition). Philadelphia, PA: Lippincott, Williams & Wilkins.

Sekhobo, J. P., L. S. Edmunds, K. Dalenius, J. Jernigan, C. F. Davis, M. Giddings, et al. (2014). Neighborhood disparities in prevalence of childhood obesity among low-income children before and after implementation of New York City child care regulations. *Prev Chronic Dis* **11**: E181.

Singh, A. S., C. Mulder, J. W. Twisk, W. van Mechelen, and M. J. Chinapaw. (2008). Tracking of childhood overweight into adulthood: a systematic review of the literature. *Obes Rev* **9**(5): 474–488.

Soubhi, H., L. Potvin, and G. Paradis (2004). Family process and parent's leisure time physical activity. *Am J Health Behav* **28**(3): 218–230.

U.S. Department of Health and Human Services. (2008). *Physical activity guidelines*. Washington, DC: Office of Disease Prevention and Health Promotion.

Ussher, M. H., A. H. Taylor, and G. E. Faulkner. (2014). Exercise interventions for smoking cessation. *Cochrane Database Syst Rev* **8**: CD002295.

Vandenbroeck, I. P., D. J. Goossens, and M. Clemens. (2007). *Tackling obesities: future choices: obesity system atlas*. London: UK Government Office for Science.

Veerman, J. L. (2011). On the futility of screening for genes that make you fat. *PLoS Med* **8**(11): e1001114.

Whitaker, R. C., J. A. Wright, M. S. Pepe, K. D. Seidel, and W. H. Dietz. (1997). Predicting obesity in young adulthood from childhood and parental obesity. *N Engl J Med* **337**(13): 869–873.

12

Case Study

SIMULATING THE IMPACT OF HIGH-RISK
AND POPULATION INTERVENTION STRATEGIES
FOR THE PREVENTION OF DISEASE

Jonathan Platt, Katherine M. Keyes, and Sandro Galea

1.0 Balancing Equity and Efficiency Through High-Risk and Population Interventions

Questions about maximizing both efficiency and equity are core considerations that inform how we may develop and implement population health interventions. As we discussed in Chapter 9, the impact of health policies and programs is often not distributed equitably throughout a population. Differences are often the result of socially embedded structures that have created historically robust, but often invisible, mechanisms through which health is determined as much by income, race, gender, or sexual orientation as it is by modifiable health behaviors (Krieger 2001). We have argued in this book that achieving equitable health distributions within populations is a central goal of population health science, as is aspiring to achieve overall improved population health. This therefore suggests that any population health intervention needs to consider both the potential impact on the whole population and also on those with different levels of risk for disease within a population and/or those in underrepresented or underserved groups. Although not always the case, the tension between equity and efficiency means that when resources are finite, there is often a tradeoff between maximizing population health while minimizing population health inequity. This balance depends on what population, disease, and risk factors are being considered, among numerous other factors (again, see Chapter 9). This ties in well with the paradigm, articulated by Geoffrey Rose more than 30 years ago, wherein interventions may focus on those deemed at high risk for disease or they may focus on disease risk throughout an entire population.

The high-risk approach seeks to identify individuals at highest risk of developing disease and to intervene to offer individual protection from developing that condition. There are two different ways this protection may be inferred. A high-risk primary prevention strategy seeks to identify high-risk individuals based on exposures known to increase the risk of developing disease significantly (i.e., risk factors) and to intervene to reduce those exposures. The goal of this strategy is to reduce the number of incident cases of disease or prevent a proportion of disease from ever occurring. An example of a high-risk intervention strategy is a program to provide counseling and/or needle exchange programs to injecting drug users to prevent incident cases of HIV, which can be transmitted through needle sharing (Watters et al. 1994, Riley and O'Hare 2000, Vlahov et al. 2010). A high-risk secondary prevention strategy seeks to identify high-risk individuals already with the disease and to reduce disease morbidity, or to decrease the prevalence of disease by shifting disease symptoms to subclinical levels. In the case of secondary prevention, the high-risk individuals often represent the most severe cases of disease, especially if risk factors of concern are strong causes of disease, or those with the least access to existing health services. An example of high-risk secondary prevention is a program to provide combination drug therapy for patients with multidrug-resistant tuberculosis (Caminero et al. 2010, WHO 2010).

In contrast, the population approach seeks to reduce the distribution of disease throughout the population as a whole. Rather than focusing on those defined as high risk, a population approach is based on implementing universal strategies, regardless of baseline risk. As with the high-risk approach, the population approach can be designed for both primary and secondary prevention. A population primary prevention strategy seeks to reduce exposure to a highly prevalent risk factor for disease. An example of this strategy is the implementation of population vaccination programs, which must be delivered to a large proportion of the population to prevent disease adequately to achieve herd immunity (Anderson and May 1985). A population secondary prevention strategy seeks to disseminate a global treatment strategy throughout an entire population to identify and/or treat cases to reduce disease morbidity. If the disease is curable, secondary prevention might also seek to cure a proportion of those with the disease. For example, it is recommended that all women begin regular breast cancer screening around middle age, with the goal of identifying extant but previously unknown cases of cancer and, through early treatment, reduce cancer mortality (Kelsey and Bernstein 1996). However, it is worth noting that, in the case of breast cancer, a movement has been made toward a high-risk strategy, given concerns about overdiagnosis and treatment from population secondary prevention programs. High-risk strategy proponents suggest women specifically with a family history of breast cancer undergo screening at younger ages (Bleyer and Welch 2012).

In summary, both high-risk and population intervention strategies can be implemented as primary prevention, which seeks to prevent the incidence of disease, and secondary prevention, which seeks to treat or cure those with disease. The main difference between strategies is who the focus of the intervention will be. The high-risk strategy is generally implemented to decrease disease inequalities and increase health equity, whereas the population strategy seeks to maximize the number of individuals reached by an intervention, with less concern for the differential risk individuals face in developing disease. As discussed in Chapter 9, these decisions are guided as much by values as by cost–benefit analyses. In this chapter we offer, by way of illustration, an analysis of which approach is optimal for maximizing population health. Central to the work presented here is an awareness of equity and efficiency tradeoffs, and it is enriched by a consideration of all approaches through the use of simulations and sensitivity analyses. To compare the impact of four strategies—high-risk primary prevention, high-risk secondary prevention, population primary prevention, population secondary prevention—we simulated multiple versions of each intervention based on empirical population-based data to understand the effects of different strategies on population prevalence and distribution of disease. In particular, we were interested in assessing whether interventions to decrease BMI and reduce smoking are associated with lower systolic blood pressure (SBP). Hypertension is a highly relevant condition in the United States because it represents a disease outcome *and* is a modifiable risk factor for many other highly prevalent diseases, such as cardiovascular disease (Kannel 1996) and stroke (Collins et al. 1990). Furthermore, hypertension is a largely symptomless condition, which has implications for intervention strategies. Namely, individuals with chronic asymptomatic conditions are less likely to present in clinical settings and are also less likely to adhere to treatment regimens compared with those with more perceptible symptoms (Miller 1997). Therefore, it is critical to understand the impact of high-risk and population prevention programs on hypertension because they inform critical public health thinking needed to reverse the incidence and course of hypertension in a population.

2.0 The Analytic Approach

Using data from the National Health and Nutrition Examination Survey (NHANES) 2011–2012, we modeled the distribution of respondents' SBP. Respondents for whom SBP data were available formed the foundation of our total population, in which we then simulated potential interventions. SBP was chosen because it is easily measured and is a fairly normally distributed continuous variable for which there is a generally accepted threshold for disease (hypertension) in the U.S. population. Although hypertension is typically defined as SBP greater than 139 mmHg (Chobanian et al. 2003), we included those with SBP greater than 130 mmHg as hypertensive to avoid unstable results resulting from small sample sizes. The impact of each intervention was generally similar using the threshold of SBP greater than 139 mmHg for hypertension. Also, although diastolic blood pressure is certainly a health concern as well, we limited the current consideration to SBP for purposes of simplicity.

The NHANES sample comprised 7053 individuals who reported at least one measure of SBP. The average SBP value was recorded among those with multiple measurements. The sample mean SBP was 118.8 mmHg and the standard deviation (SD) was 18.4. However, to reduce the influence of extremely high or low SBP measures, we excluded individuals who reported an SBP greater than 2 SDs outside the entire population distribution. Similarly, to avoid the potential selection bias from very young or very old study participants, we limited our analytic sample to those age 25 to 65 years ($n = 3393$). The mean SBP in this sample was 119.6 ± 13.7 (Figure 12.1).

Next, we identified two exposures in the population positively associated with increased blood pressure and incident hypertension (Chobanian et al. 2003): high BMI (Wilson et al. 2002, Hall 2003) and tobacco smoking (Sleight 1993). Current smoking was defined as self-reported use of tobacco every day or some days during the past 30 days. BMI, calculated as a ratio of weight to height (kilograms per square meter), was measured by trained health technicians as a part of the standard NHANES interview protocol. General clinical BMI cut points were as follows: BMI <18.5, underweight; BMI 18.5–24.99, normal weight; BMI 25.0–29.99, overweight; BMI >30.0, obese (National Heart, Lung and Blood Institute 1998). High BMI was defined as a BMI of 25 or greater. These two exposures were chosen as illustrative because they represent a common (high BMI) and a less common (tobacco smoking) exposure in the population, and are also both considered modifiable risk behaviors in the population (Lackland 2005). That is, there are numerous interventions through which individuals can reduce their BMI or quit smoking. Both risk

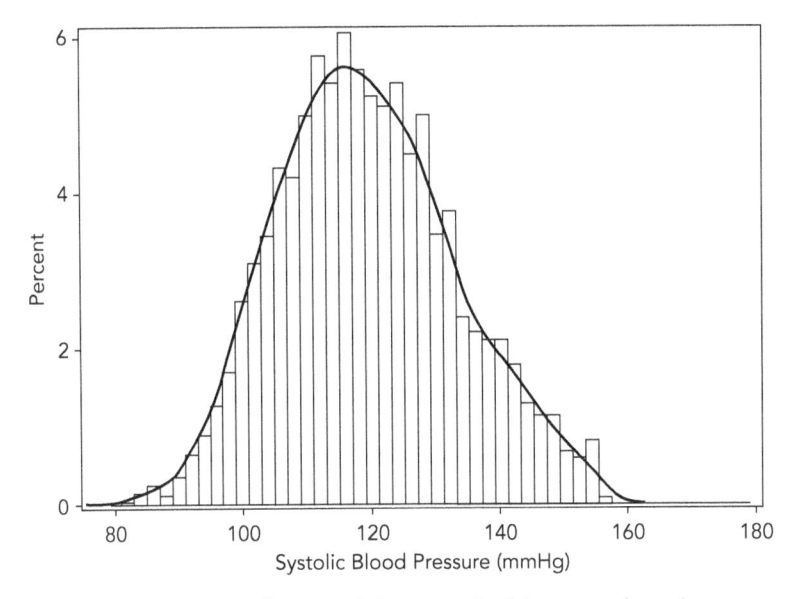

FIGURE 12.1 Distribution of SBP in adults ±2 standard deviations from the total sample mean of individuals age 25–65 in the National Health and Nutrition Examination Survey 2011–2012 (n = 3393).

factor prevalence and how an intervention is defined (Hernan and Taubman 2008) are important considerations in guiding intervention strategies. For simplicity, overweight and obese categories were combined into one "high BMI" category compared with those with a BMI less than 25.

Mean SBP increased as clinical BMI classification increased, from 111.4 mmHg among underweight individuals to 123.3 mmHg among severely obese individuals. Also, the prevalence of hypertension increased with BMI, from 12.8% among underweight to 29.6% among severely obese. Similar patterns were seen with smoking status. Compared with nonsmokers, smokers' SBP was 2 mmHg higher, and the prevalence of hypertension increased from 19.3% to 22.4%. The SD was not substantially different for any risk factor category except among the underweight group, although this is likely a result of the small sample size (Table 12.1).

Using these data as a starting place, we simulated the effects of each intervention strategy based on the hypothetical manipulation of the distributions of BMI, smoking, and/or SBP.

For high-risk primary prevention, we defined those individuals who reported both current smoking and high BMI as high risk (n = 495). To examine the effect of the high-risk primary prevention strategy, we simulated the change in SBP distribution as a result of, hypothetically, removing one

Table 12.1 Prevalence of High BMI and Current Smoking in the General Population Shows Higher SBP with Increased BMI and among Smokers

Population Characteristic	n (%)	Mean SBP, mmHg	SBP SD, mmHg	SBP > 130 mmHg, n (%)
BMI status				
Any high BMI (>25)	2348 (69.0)	121.1	13.3	558 (23.8)
Underweight (<18.5)	47 (1.4)	111.4	17.2	6 (12.8)
Normal weight (18.5–24.99)	983 (29.3)	116.1	13.7	152 (15.5)
Overweight (25–29.99)	1108 (33.0)	120.0	13.1	221 (20.0)
Obese (30–34.99)	670 (20.0)	121.3	13.1	168 (25.1)
Severely obese (>35)	548 (16.3)	123.3	13.6	162 (29.6)
Smoking status				
Current smoker	765 (23.0)	120.4	13.7	171 (22.4)
Not a current smoker	1941 (77.0)	118.4	13.8	374 (19.3)

BMI, body mass index; SBP, systolic blood pressure; SD, standard deviation.

risk factor from the high-risk population. To simulate the effect of smoking prevention, we reduced the SBP of each individual in the high-risk population by the mean difference between the population who reported smoking (SBP = 120.4 mmHg) and the population who reported not smoking (SBP = 118.4 mmHg). To simulate the effect of prevention of high BMI among the high-risk group, we reduced the SBP of each individual by the mean difference in SBP between high (SBP = 121.1 mmHg) and normal (SBP = 116 mmHg) BMI groups. For simplicity, we assumed the risk factors were independent and were associated linearly with SBP.

For high-risk secondary prevention, because secondary prevention usually implies clinical treatment, we defined the high-risk population as individuals with an average SBP of 130 mmHg or more. We modeled two different strategies to simulate the effect of treating high-risk individuals using clinical approaches. In strategy A, we measured changes in SBP distribution as a result of treatment to reduce the SBP of high-risk individuals to 130 mmHg, 125 mmHg, and 120 mmHg. In strategy B, we repeated the steps from the first high-risk treatment approach, except we simulated the effect of reducing the SBP of high-risk hypertensive individuals by 5%, 10%, and 15% to simulate an intervention that focuses on high-risk group-level percentage decreases, rather than targeted decreases in individual-level BMI. For both secondary prevention strategies, we examined the sensitivity of intervention intensiveness by simulating three reasonable SBP reduction goals that might be devised between a high-risk individual and a physician.

For population primary prevention, we simulated changes in the SBP distribution assuming a hypothetical reduction of mean BMI and smoking throughout the entire population. We modeled the distribution of SBP assuming a BMI reduction of 10% and 25%, and a reduction in the prevalence of smoking by 33% and 50%. To do this, we calculated the mean SBP difference for every 1-unit change in BMI in the population (e.g., <18.5, 18.5–19.49, 19.5–20.49, . . . >45.5). Next, we decreased each individual's BMI by 10%. We imputed their adjusted SBP, based on the difference between the mean SBP of their reported BMI and the mean SBP of their 10% decreased BMI. We then repeated these steps, assuming a 25% decrease in population BMI. For smoking prevention, we randomly selected 33% of the population who were current smokers and imputed their adjusted SBP as the mean SBP of the nonsmoking population. We repeated these steps for 50% of the smoking population. Using this strategy, all reductions were made randomly in the population, independent of other risk factors or baseline SBP that individuals reported.

For population secondary prevention, we simulated the changes in the distribution of SBP if hypertensive individuals in the general population were targeted, regardless of risk factors, to achieve reductions of 2.5%, 5%, and 10%. As in the high-risk treatment approaches, we used different levels of reduction to simulate varying levels of intensiveness of the intervention targets.

In addition, we measured the baseline SBP distributions in several sociodemographic groups for which there is a known disparity in hypertension prevalence. Specifically, we modeled the SBP distribution stratified by the lowest and highest recorded levels of annual household income (Diez-Roux et al. 2000) (<$35,000 vs. >$100,000, respectively), and non-Hispanic white versus non-Hispanic black race (Hertz et al. 2005). SBP distribution for each group was modeled separately, and race and income groups were combined to model the distribution of risk factors and the distribution of SBP among subgroups in a general population with well-known hypertension inequalities. We then simulated each of the four interventions among the low- and high-income subpopulations as a way to examine their impact in groups with a different baseline risk of disease, and to examine the extent to which visible behavioral risk factors were attributable to hypertension inequalities.

For each of these simulated interventions, we calculated the mean, SD, prevalence, and absolute number of cases of hypertension in each population. Each of these measures allow us to investigate distinct aspects of the interventions.

The mean allows us to see the overall center of blood pressure for the subset of the population, given its exposure. Comparing changes in the population mean shows the overall population effect of each intervention.

Comparing the SD around the mean SBP allows us to see the proportion of individuals in the upper and lower bounds of the SBP distribution. For the purposes of this simulation, we are particularly interested in those individuals in the upper bounds of the SBP distribution, which is indicative of cases of hypertension. By calculating the percent change in prevalence of hypertension, we can assess the relative clinical effectiveness of one intervention strategy versus others. We can also calculate the number of cases reduced, given an intervention, as an absolute measure of change in disease prevalence in the population. The SD, combined with the changes in hypertension prevalence, allows us to start to examine the effect of each intervention in decreasing population SBP inequalities. One particular intervention may reduce the population mean SBP, which suggests that it would have the effect of decreasing the prevalence of the outcome for the entire sample. However, comparing the relative decreases in the standard deviation and prevalence of hypertension for each intervention would highlight the degree to which an intervention might decrease the proportion of the sample in the upper bounds of SBP distribution, or those with the greatest need of the intervention.

As a way to examine the absolute effects of each intervention visually, and the effects relative to other interventions, we standardized the SBP values for each individual to a normal distribution using the resulting population mean and SD after each intervention. We plotted the SBP distributions, comparing the effects of high-risk primary and secondary prevention strategies in Figure 12.1, and population primary and secondary prevention strategies in Figure 12.2.

3.0 The Effects of Interventions on Population Distributions of SBP and the Prevalence of High Blood Pressure

3.1 High-Risk Prevention Interventions

First, we examined the effects of the high-risk prevention strategy. The mean SBP among the high-risk population was 121.6 mmHg, two points greater than that of the general population. The effect of primary prevention decreased the SBP mean and SD to 119.2 ± 12.68 mmHg and 118.7 ± 12.73 mmHg

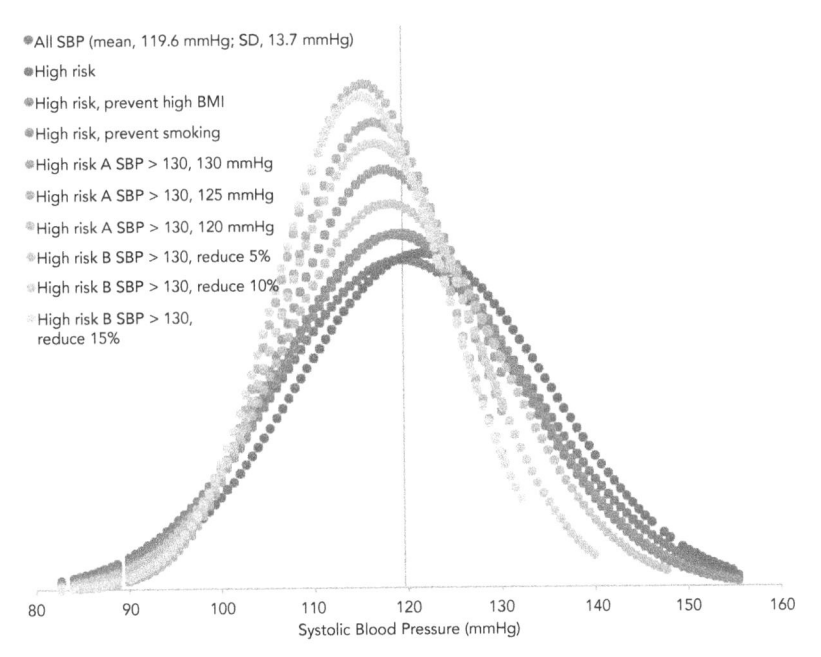

Legend (top-left of figure):
- All SBP (mean, 119.6 mmHg; SD, 13.7 mmHg)
- High risk
- High risk, prevent high BMI
- High risk, prevent smoking
- High risk A SBP > 130, 130 mmHg
- High risk A SBP > 130, 125 mmHg
- High risk A SBP > 130, 120 mmHg
- High risk B SBP > 130, reduce 5%
- High risk B SBP > 130, reduce 10%
- High risk B SBP > 130, reduce 15%

FIGURE 12.2 Systolic blood pressure (SBP) distribution in the general population and the high-risk population, and subsequent changes resulting from high-risk primary and secondary prevention strategies. High-risk intervention A targeted only those at high risk defined as those individuals who reported both smoking and high body mass index (BMI; $n = 495$). High-risk intervention B targeted only those at high risk defined as those individuals whose SBP was greater than 130 mmHg ($n = 719$). SD, standard deviation.

for smoking and high-BMI prevention, respectively. Large reductions in mean SBP were seen in both secondary prevention strategies. The largest decrease was 115.1 mmHg, after high-risk SBP was reduced by 15%, but the narrowest SD (8.9 mmHg) occurred when high-risk individuals achieved an SBP reduction to 120 mmHg. Compared with the general population, strategy A reduced 100% of the prevalence of hypertension and strategy B reduced 95.8% of hypertension. Compared with the baseline high-risk population, the most intensive versions of secondary prevention A and B achieved 100% and 96.3% reductions in hypertension prevalence, respectively. All high-risk strategy results can be examined in Table 12.2 and in Figure 12.2.

As shown in Table 12.2, among high-risk strategies, secondary prevention strategy B led to the greatest decrease in SBP mean whereas secondary prevention strategy A led to the greatest decreases in SPB SD and prevalence of hypertension in the general population ($n = 3393$).

In summary, the high-risk prevention strategies A and B both led to significant decreases in SBP mean, SD, as well as cases of hypertension, although

Table 12.2 Mean SBP, SD, and Changes in Cases under Hypothetical High-Risk Intervention Scenarios

Population Characteristics	n (%)	Mean SBP, mmHg	SBP SD, mmHg	SBP > 130 mmHg, n (%)	Change in Cases[a] vs. Population, n (%)	Change in Cases[a] vs. High Risk,[b] n (%)
Population SBP	3393	119.6	13.7	719 (21.2)	—	—
High-risk SBP	495 (14.6)	121.6	13.4	121 (24.4)	(13.1)	—
High risk, primary prevention[b]						
Prevent smoking	3393	119.2	12.7	598 (17.6)	−121 (−17.0)	(−27.9)
Prevent high BMI	3393	118.7	12.7	598 (17.6)	−121 (−17.0)	(−27.9)
High risk, secondary prevention A[c]						
Reduce SBP to 130 mmHg	3393	117.6	10.7	0 (0.0)	−719 (−100.0)	(−100.0)
Reduce SBP to 125 mmHg	3393	116.5	9.7	0 (0.0)	−719 (−100.0)	(−100.0)
Reduce SBP to 120 mmHg	3393	115.5	8.9	0 (0.0)	−719 (−100.0)	(−100.0)
High risk, secondary prevention B[c]						
Reduce SBP 5%	3393	118.1	11.1	401 (11.8)	−318 (−44.3)	(−51.6)
Reduce SBP 10%	3393	116.6	10.1	167 (4.9)	−552 (−76.9)	(−79.9)
Reduce SBP 15%	3393	115.1	9.1	31 (0.9)	−688 (−95.8)	(−96.3)

BMI, body mass index; SD, standard deviation; SBP, systolic blood pressure.
[a] Cases of hypertension defined as those with an SBP greater than 130 mmHg.
[b] The intervention targeted only those at high risk, defined as those individuals who reported both smoking and high BMI (n = 495).
[c] The intervention targeted only those at high risk, defined as those individuals whose SBP was greater than 130 mmHg (n = 719).

the SBP mean decrease was slightly greater in strategy B. The impact of primary prevention did little to decrease SBP mean and SD, although it did lead to a meaningful decrease in hypertension prevalence.

3.2 Population Prevention

Next we examined the results of both population prevention strategies. As a result of primary prevention strategies, a reduction of high BMI by 10% and 25% decreased SBP to 119.4 mmHg and 119.0 mmHg, respectively. Reducing smoking levels by 33% and 50% only reduced mean SBP to 119.4 mmHg and 119.3 mmHg, respectively. Similarly, no primary prevention strategies reduced population SDs, and the 10% high BMI reduction even resulted in 25 more cases of hypertension (a 3.3% relative increase). The impact of reducing the population of smokers by 50% prevented nine cases of hypertension (1.4%) in the general population. The secondary prevention strategy achieved substantial decreases in the population SBP mean and SD. An 8% reduction in population SBP decreased the overall mean SBP by 4.8 mmHg to 114.8 ± 9.7 mmHg. The prevalence of hypertension decreased by 25.0%, 44.3%, and 64.2%, as a result of 2.5%, 5%, and 8% changes, respectively, from population secondary prevention strategies. That primary prevention increased the prevalence of hypertension slightly in the population was an unexpected finding, although it may be a result of nonsignificant fluctuations in hypertension prevalence. Recall that the mean SBP was calculated for every 1-unit change in BMI and was imputed based on the adjusted BMI (after a 10% or 25% reduction). For example, a 10% decrease in BMI from 26.5 to 23.85 led to a corresponding increase in SBP by 0.99 mmHg. The population strategy results can be examined in Table 12.3 and in Figure 12.3.

As seen in Table 12.3, among population strategies, primary prevention had little impact whereas secondary prevention led to substantial decreases in SBP mean, SD, and prevalence of hypertension in the general population ($n = 3393$).

In summary, primary prevention strategies did little to change the population distribution of SBP and hypertension, whereas the secondary prevention strategy led to decreases in SBP mean, SD, and hypertension prevalence that increased at every level of intervention intensiveness.

3.3 Population Inequalities in SBP and Risk Factors by Race and Income

We examined inequalities in SBP distribution by two races and two income groups. The SBP mean and SD were significantly greater among non-Hispanic

Table 12.3 Mean SBP, SD, and Changes in Cases under Hypothetical Population Intervention Scenarios

Population Characteristics	Mean SBP, mmHg	SBP SD, mmHg	SBP > 130 mmHg, n (%)	Change in Cases vs. Population, n (%)
Population SBP	119.6	13.7	719 (21.2)	—
Population primary prevention[a]				
Reduce high BMI 10%	119.4	13.8	744 (21.9)	25 (3.3)
Reduce high BMI 25%	119.0	13.8	715 (21.1)	−4 (−0.5)
Reduce smoking 33%	119.4	13.7	712 (21.0)	−7 (−0.9)
Reduce smoking by 50%	119.3	13.7	710 (20.9)	−9 (−1.4)
Population secondary prevention[b]				
Reduce SBP 2.5%	118.1	12.3	540 (15.9)	−179 (−25.0)
Reduce SBP 5%	116.6	11.1	401 (11.8)	−318 (−44.3)
Reduce SBP 8%	114.8	9.7	257 (7.6)	−462 (−64.2)

BMI, body mass index; SD, standard deviation; SBP, systolic blood pressure.
[a] Cases of hypertension defined as those with an SBP greater than 130 mmHg.
[b] The intervention targeted all individuals in the population, regardless of risk.

black individuals (123.3 ± 14.2 mmHg), compared with non-Hispanic white individuals (118.8 ± 12.9 mmHg). Also, the prevalence of hypertension was greater among non-Hispanic blacks (31.3%) compared with non-Hispanic whites (18.0%). The mean SBP in the low-income population was 2 mmHg greater than the high-income group (120.3 mmHg and 118.3 mmHg, respectively). The prevalence of hypertension was 22.5% and 17.8% among low- and high-income groups, respectively. Among the combined groups, the mean SBP was highest in the low-income non-Hispanic black population (122.8 ± 14.7 mmHg) and was lowest in the high-income non-Hispanic white population (118.7 ± 13.2 mmHg). Also worth noting, the mean SBP among high-income non-Hispanic blacks (121.8 mmHg) was nearly 2 points greater than in low-income non-Hispanic whites (119.7 mmHg).

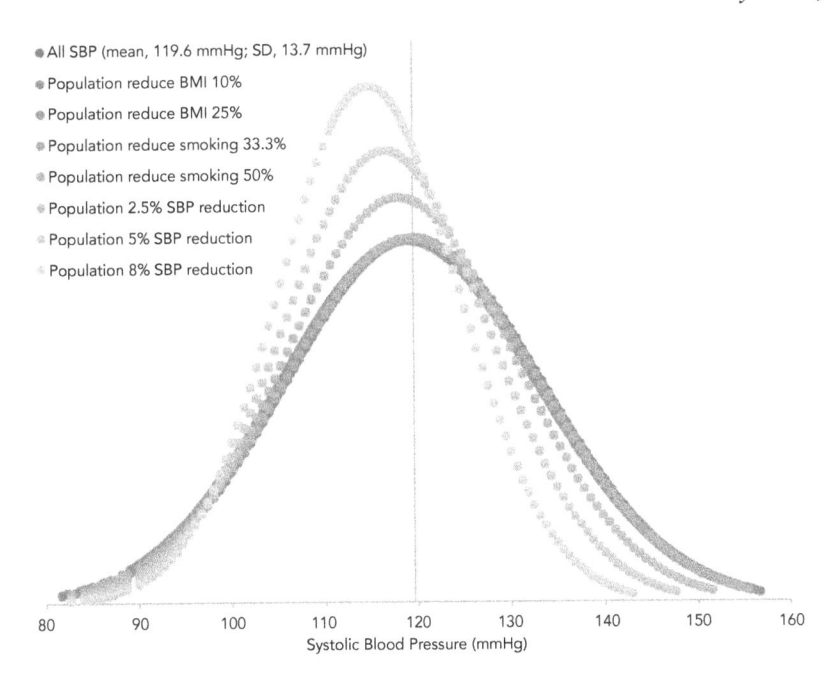

- All SBP (mean, 119.6 mmHg; SD, 13.7 mmHg)
- Population reduce BMI 10%
- Population reduce BMI 25%
- Population reduce smoking 33.3%
- Population reduce smoking 50%
- Population 2.5% SBP reduction
- Population 5% SBP reduction
- Population 8% SBP reduction

FIGURE 12.3 Systolic blood pressure (SBP) distribution in the general population showing changes as a result of population primary and secondary prevention strategies. Population intervention strategies targeted all individuals in the population, regardless of risk. BMI, body mass index; SD, standard deviation.

We contrasted these results with a closer look at the mean number of risk factors (i.e., high BMI and current smoking). The general population reported a mean of 0.92 risk factor, and 14.6% of the population was high risk, endorsing both risk factors. The low-income population reported a greater mean number of risk factors than the high-income population (1.04 vs. 0.73). Although the mean risk factors were slightly greater among the non-Hispanic black population (1.02) compared with non-Hispanic whites (0.99), the proportion of high-risk individuals was greater among non-Hispanic whites (18.5%) compared with non-Hispanic blacks (15.6%). Among the low-income non-Hispanic white population, 30.4% were high risk compared with only 2.5% of high-income non-Hispanic blacks.

To summarize, SBP inequalities were observed within both income and race groups, in which low-income and non-Hispanic black groups showed greater mean SBP and hypertension prevalence than their high-income, non-Hispanic white counterparts. It is questionable whether these inequalities are attributable to the risk factors in our study.

3.4 The Effects of Prevention Strategies in Low-Household Income and High-Household Income Populations

We simulated the effects of each intervention in a sample stratified by low- and high-income individuals to examine the impact of interventions in different socioeconomic contexts. The proportion of high-risk individuals was much higher in the low-income (21.1%) compared with the high-income (7.4%) group. The reduction in hypertension prevalence achieved through high-risk primary prevention in the low-income population was nearly three times greater than the high-income population (23.1% vs. 8.1%). The greatest reduction in SD was achieved by the high-risk secondary prevention A strategy, which was 8.8 mmHg in the low-income group and 9.0 mmHg in the high-income group distributions. The impact of population primary prevention strategies was minimal in both populations and, similar to the results in the general population, led to increases in the prevalence of hypertension among those who remained as "high BMI" in both income groups, after 10% and 25% BMI reductions. Both the high-risk and the population secondary prevention strategies achieved substantial decreases in mean SBP and hypertension prevalence. The most intensive level of high-risk secondary prevention decreased the mean SBP to 115.6 ± 9.1 mmHg in the low-income population and 114.6 ± 9.1 mmHg among the high-income population, whereas the most intensive level of population secondary prevention decreased the mean SBP to 115.3 ± 9.8 mmHg in the low-income population and 114.0 ± 9.3 mmHg in the high-income population. The corresponding reductions in baseline hypertension achieved by the 8% reduction in SBP were 62.2% in the low-income group and 65.2% in the high-income group. Key differences in interventions between income groups are summarized in Table 12.4.

In summary, the lowest postintervention levels of mean SBP were seen among the high-income population, although this is, in part, because the baseline SBP was lower than the low-income group. Relative to baseline levels, the greatest SBP reductions were seen in the low-income group. The impact of high-risk primary prevention led to greater decreases in hypertension prevalence among the low-income population whereas the impact of population secondary prevention led to slightly greater decreases in hypertension prevalence among the high-income population.

Table 12.4 Summary of Effects of Hypothetical Intervention Strategies among High and Low Household Income Earners

Intervention Strategy	Low Household Income (<$35,000/y)	High Household Income (>$100,000/y)	Overall
High risk			
Primary prevention	Larger decrease in SD and hypertension prevalence		No significant reductions in mean SBP for either group
Secondary prevention A	Larger decrease in mean SBP		Reductions in SD and hypertension prevalence not different by income group
Secondary prevention B	Larger decrease in mean SBP	Larger decrease in hypertension prevalence	Reductions in SD not different by income group
Population			
Primary prevention			No significant reductions in SBP mean, SD, or hypertension prevalence
Secondary prevention	Larger decrease in mean SBP	Larger decrease in SBP SD and hypertension prevalence	

SD, standard deviation; SBP, systolic blood pressure.

4.0 Summary: Population and High-Risk Strategies for Reducing Blood Pressure in the Population

Each of the four different intervention strategies modeled had a distinct impact on the SBP mean, distribution, and prevalence of hypertension in the study population. The greatest reductions in mean SBP resulted from the population secondary prevention, whereas the greatest reductions in SBP SD resulted from the high-risk secondary prevention strategy A. Compared with the baseline, secondary prevention achieved a greater decrease in hypertension prevalence in the high-risk population than in the general population. The effect of reducing the prevalence of high BMI and current smoking in both primary prevention strategies did very little to decrease population mean and SD, although it did lead to a 17% decrease in the prevalence of hypertension when prevention efforts targeted high-risk individuals.

Stratifying by low and high household income highlighted important differences in each strategy. The high-risk primary prevention strategy decreased the prevalence of hypertension among low-income individuals by almost one quarter (23.1%), whereas the impact was less than 10% among the high-income population. In our population, recall that the mean number of risk factors in the low-income population was 1.04 ± 0.62 and was 0.73 ± 0.59 in the high-income population. Therefore, it makes intuitive sense that those with a greater number of risk factors (i.e., those with low income) stand to gain more from efforts to reduce the prevalence of those exposures.

On the other hand, the SBP distribution among black individuals compared with white individuals did not follow this pattern. The mean numbers of risk factors between these two groups were much more similar (1.02 ± 0.54 vs. 0.99 ± 0.61 for black and white individuals, respectively). By the logic of the income gradient, we would expect to see their associated SBP means to be similar as well. In our sample, however, the mean SBP was 4.5 mmHg higher among blacks (123.3 mmHg) and the prevalence of hypertension was 1.74 times higher compared with whites. This finding is a result of at least two social patterns not investigated in this case study. First, white individuals, through social stratification, are generally more likely to earn a higher income and thus are more likely to receive the health benefits conferred by greater economic resources (Deaton and Lubotsky 2003). In our sample, in an unweighted analysis, 24.2% of whites and 14.2% of blacks reported being "high income" (data not shown). Second, there are undoubtedly many other risk factors for hypertension in addition to smoking and high BMI. Minority populations have a historically greater risk of chronic health conditions resulting from many of the same reasons underlying the income–health gradient, and often face discriminatory experiences, an additional risk factor for hypertension (Pamuk 1998, Williams and Mohammed 2009). A thorough investigation of racial inequalities in chronic health is beyond the scope of this chapter, but we bring it up here to emphasize the point that a researcher or clinician who chooses to define a high-risk population based solely on the prevalence of "modifiable" risk factors (i.e., smoking and high BMI) would overlook significant causes of inequalities in health outcomes.

A high-risk population can be defined by any number of criteria. One may choose a definition based on sociodemographic groups such as age, sex, race/ethnicity, income, or neighborhood, or high risk may be defined using "modifiable" risk behaviors, such as smoking, physical activity, substance use, or other comorbid conditions. There is not always a clear distinction between what is or is not modifiable (e.g., social isolation [Berkman et al. 2003, Pantell et al. 2013]). For these reasons, it is important to consider the assumptions and implications of how we define who is at high risk. Focusing on what is modifiable may allow for a more well-defined intervention, but it may lead one to address the most proximate causes of disease, rather than thinking about risk in terms of macrosocial or structural determinants.

A more general but related limitation of the high-risk approach, as discussed by Rose (1985), and as illustrated in this book in Chapter 10, is the difficulty we face in predicting individual risk for disease. In our simulations, despite modeling two well-established risk factors for hypertension, the act of reducing the prevalence of individual exposure to smoking and high BMI did little to reduce the overall population mean SBP, especially when primary prevention was attempted for the entire population. As the underlying risk in the high-risk population increased, so, too, did the efficacy of the primary prevention strategies (e.g., in the general vs. low-income population). The efficacy of these strategies for an individual is limited by our ability to predict the individual risk of disease, which illustrates our sixth foundational principle (the magnitude of the effect of an exposure on disease is dependent on the prevalence of the causal factors that interact with that exposure), which leads directly to the ninth foundational principle (we can predict health in populations with much more certainty than we can predict health in individuals). The magnitude of the effect of an exposure on disease is dependent on the prevalence of the causal factors that interact with that exposure. We will improve our ability to predict an individual's risk for disease by understanding how multiple risk factors interact to cause disease. Our predictive ability might also increase by defining our high-risk population in more narrow terms (e.g., low-income individuals who report smoking and a high BMI), but we do so knowing that the absolute number of cases we can prevent will likely decrease as the population becomes smaller. For example, the primary prevention strategy decreased hypertension among low-income individuals by 23.1% versus 17% in the general population. However, the general population was comprised of 3393 individuals, so a decrease of 17% prevented 121 cases of hypertension, whereas the low-income population was comprised of 1358 individuals, so a decrease of 23.1% prevented only 70 cases of hypertension. In addition, high-risk strategies imply that high-risk individuals must be identified and consent to participating in an intervention, both of which are difficult and expensive.

In contrast, population strategies focus on universal strategies that impact all individuals, regardless of baseline risk. This universality has advantages and disadvantages. A population strategy typically seeks to decrease population-level risk of disease, which is why vaccination programs strive for herd immunity by maximizing population coverage of vaccines. At the individual level, most individuals would never get the disease with or without the vaccination. As mentioned earlier, Rose (1985) referred to this as the "prevention paradox." This can make the implementation of a population-level intervention difficult, especially in the short term. Indeed, recent calls to increase the tax on sugar-sweetened beverages in New York City were met with staunch resistance and were, ultimately, defeated, in part because opponents believed beverage choice was an individual decision, and the risk conferred by high-fructose corn syrup is not perceived as worth the increased cost by the individual consumer (Brownell et al. 2009, Gollust et al. 2014). When they do succeed, however, population strategies can be powerfully sustainable drivers of healthy behavior change. For example, workplace smoking bans have been shown to encourage smokers to quit or to reduce tobacco consumption (Fichtenberg and Glantz 2002).

The simulation also illustrates our fifth foundational principle—namely, small changes in ubiquitous causes result in more substantial change in the health of populations than larger changes in rarer causes. This can be seen to a small degree in the difference in reducing high BMI, a highly prevalent (69.0%) exposure, compared with the effect of reducing smoking, a relatively less prevalent exposure (23.0%) in our population. Because of this, a 25% reduction in population BMI achieved a greater reduction in mean SBP than a 50% reduction in smoking in the population.

In conclusion, each of the four different intervention strategies had a distinct impact on the SBP mean, distribution, and prevalence of hypertension in the study population. The greatest reductions in mean SBP resulted from the population secondary prevention whereas the greatest reductions in SBP SD resulted from high-risk secondary prevention strategy A. Compared with the baseline, secondary prevention achieved a greater decrease in hypertension prevalence in the high-risk population than in the general population. The effect of reducing the prevalence of high BMI and current smoking in both primary prevention strategies did little to decrease population SBP mean and SD, although it did lead to a 17% decrease in the prevalence of hypertension when prevention efforts targeted high-risk individuals.

We end by restating our eighth foundational principle: efforts to improve overall population health may be a disadvantage to some groups; whether equity or efficiency is preferable is a matter of values. These values are influential in every step of the process of intervening to improve population health. Our collective biases, judgments, and goals determine the specific types and targets of any intervention, as well as which parameters we include (or exclude) and how they are estimated. These values must be made transparent when designing a quantitative intervention for population health impact.

5.0 References

Anderson, R. M., and R. M. May. (1985). Vaccination and herd immunity to infectious diseases. *Nature* **318**(6044): 323–329.

Berkman, L. F., J. Blumenthal, M. Burg, R. M. Carney, D. Catellier, M. J. Cowan, et al. (2003). Effects of treating depression and low perceived social support on clinical events after myocardial infarction: the Enhancing Recovery in Coronary Heart Disease Patients (ENRICHD) Randomized Trial. *JAMA* **289**(23): 3106–3116.

Bleyer, A., and H. G. Welch. (2012). Effect of three decades of screening mammography on breast-cancer incidence. *N Engl J Med* **367**(21): 1998–2005.

Brownell, K. D., T. Farley, W. C. Willett, B. M. Popkin, F. J. Chaloupka, J. W. Thompson, et al. (2009). The public health and economic benefits of taxing sugar-sweetened beverages. *N Engl J Med* **361**(16): 1599–1605.

Caminero, J. A., G. Sotgiu, A. Zumla, and G. B. Migliori. (2010). Best drug treatment for multidrug-resistant and extensively drug-resistant tuberculosis. *Lancet Infect Dis* **10**(9): 621–629.

Chobanian, A. V., G. L. Bakris, H. R. Black, W. C. Cushman, L. A. Green, J. L. Izzo, et al. (2003). Seventh report of the Joint National Committee on Prevention, Detection, Evaluation, and Treatment of High Blood Pressure. *Hypertension* **42**(6): 1206–1252.

Collins, R., R. Peto, S. MacMahon, J. Godwin, N. Qizilbash, P. Hebert, et al. (1990). Blood pressure, stroke, and coronary heart disease: part 2: short-term reductions in blood pressure: overview of randomised drug trials in their epidemiological context. *Lancet* **335**(8693): 827–838.

Deaton, A., and D. Lubotsky. (2003). Mortality, inequality and race in American cities and states. *Soc Sci Med* **56**(6): 1139–1153.

Diez-Roux, A. V., B. G. Link, and M. E. Northridge. (2000). A multilevel analysis of income inequality and cardiovascular disease risk factors. *Soc Sci Med* **50**(5): 673–687.

Fichtenberg, C. M., and S. A. Glantz. (2002). Effect of smoke-free workplaces on smoking behaviour: systematic review. *BMJ* **325**(7357): 188.

Gollust, S. E., C. L. Barry, and J. Niederdeppe. (2014). Americans' opinions about policies to reduce consumption of sugar-sweetened beverages. *Prev Med* **63**: 52–57.

Hall, J. E. (2003). The kidney, hypertension, and obesity. *Hypertension* **41**(3): 625–633.

Hernan, M. A., and S. L. Taubman. (2008). Does obesity shorten life? The importance of well-defined interventions to answer causal questions. *Int J Obes (Lond)* **32**(Suppl 3): S8–S14.

Hertz, R. P., A. N. Unger, J. A. Cornell, and E. Saunders. (2005). Racial disparities in hypertension prevalence, awareness, and management. *Arch Intern Med* **165**(18): 2098–2104.

Kannel, W. B. (1996). Blood pressure as a cardiovascular risk factor: prevention and treatment. *JAMA* **275**(20): 1571–1576.

Kelsey, J. L., and L. Bernstein. (1996). Epidemiology and prevention of breast cancer. *Annu Review Public Health* **17**(1): 47–67.

Krieger, N. (2001). Theories for social epidemiology in the 21st century: an ecosocial perspective. *Int J Epidemiol* **30**(4): 668–677.

Lackland, D. T. (2005). Population strategies to treat hypertension. *Curr Treat Options Cardiovasc Med* **7**(4): 253–258.

Miller, N. H. (1997). Compliance with treatment regimens in chronic asymptomatic diseases. *Am J Med* **102**(2): 43–49.

National Institutes of Health, National Heart, Lung, and Blood Institute. (1998). Clinical guidelines on the identification, evaluation, and treatment of overweight and obesity in adults; the evidence report. *Obes Res* **6**(suppl 2): 51–209S.

Pamuk E., D. Makuc, K. Heck, C. Reuben, K. Lochner. (1998). Socioeconomic Status and Health Chartbook: Health, United States. Hyattsville, Maryland: National Center for Health Statistics.

Pantell, M., D. Rehkopf, D. Jutte, S. L. Syme, J. Balmes, and N. Adler. (2013). Social isolation: a predictor of mortality comparable to traditional clinical risk factors. *Am J Public Health* **103**(11): 2056–2062.

Riley, D., and P. O'Hare. (2000). Harm reduction: history, definition, and practice. *Harm Reduct Natl Int Perspect* **1000**: 1–26.

Rose, G. (1985). Sick individuals and sick populations. *Int J Epidemiol* **20**(30): 427–432.

Sleight, P. (1993). Smoking and hypertension. *Clin Exp Hypertens* **15**(6): 1181–1192.

Vlahov, D., A. M. Robertson, and S. A. Strathdee. (2010). Prevention of HIV infection among injection drug users in resource-limited settings. *Clin Infect Dis* **50**(Suppl. 3): S114–S121.

Watters, J. K., M. J. Estilo, G. L. Clark, and J. Lorvick. (1994). Syringe and needle exchange as HIV/AIDS prevention for injection drug users. *JAMA* **271**(2): 115–120.

Williams, D. R., and S. A. Mohammed. (2009). Discrimination and racial disparities in health: evidence and needed research. *J Behav Med* **32**(1): 20–47.

Wilson, P. W., R. B. D'Agostino, L. Sullivan, H. Parise, and W. B. Kannel. (2002). Overweight and obesity as determinants of cardiovascular risk: the Framingham experience. *Arch Int Med* **162**(16): 1867–1872.

World Health Organization. (2010). WHO global report: Global tuberculosis control. Geneva: World Health Organization.

13

Tensions in Population Health Science

1.0 Combining Foundational Principles with Rapidly Developing Science

Throughout this book we made the case that population health science is, at its core, concerned with the distributions of health within and across populations. We suggest, therefore, that population health science is about negotiating two goals: using data and resources maximally in ways that improve health overall, and reducing health gaps in ways that achieve the goals of equity and social justice.

We argued that our aspirations to produce healthier populations require an alignment of our values and those aspirations as we aim to engage prevention and intervention efforts aimed at maximizing public good. Furthermore, we suggested that we would be well served to conduct our science explicitly with the intention of engaging questions consequential to improving the health of populations. To inform this effort, we organized this book around a series of foundational principles of population health science that focus on both content and methods. The principles can be applied to the development of theory around the drivers of population health, the design of studies that test and expand such theories, the analysis of data to uncover causal architecture, and the critical evaluation of the tradeoffs of potential prevention and intervention efforts with an eye toward improving population health. We advocated for an approach that places macrosocial determinants of health at the forefront of scientific inquiry, acknowledges the causal architecture that

---

Note: Portions of the text in this chapter are adapted from: Keyes, K. M., and S. Galea. (2016). Setting the agenda for a new discipline: population health science. *American Journal of Public Health* **106**(4): 633–634. http://www.ncbi.nlm.nih.gov/pubmed/26959265

underlies causal effects, suggests that general "risk factor" approaches are insufficient for population health science, and pursues prevention and intervention efforts focused on the nexus of return on health investment, efficiency, and health equity for all. We argued that if we think about populations centrally as part of every step of the research process, all our methods and theories will emerge from that central starting point.

Although we hope the principles articulated here stand the test of time, we recognize that science changes constantly, as it should. At this writing we find ourselves in an era of rapidly developing science and technology that allows us increasingly to collect vast amounts of individual data on populations, from biological samples taken throughout the life course to clinical records that are more and more in depth and comprehensive. As these new developments unfold, population health science has a strong role in this new era to shape questions, provide analytic guidance, and set the parameters for discussion and debate. Informed by these changes, in this chapter we review three major innovations in the way in which science is being conducted currently, and we discuss the role of population health science in each of them: the rise and promise of "big data" techniques, precision medicine, and population approaches to brain imaging and neuroscience. We are certain these are not the only three changes that matter and you, a few years hence, may find other emerging directions in the field compelling, provoking you to challenge our foundational principles. However, in tackling these three emerging areas we aim to illustrate the adaptability of our foundational principles, providing a road map for your application of these principles to other areas where science moves in coming years.

2.0   The Rise of "Big Data": Where Does Population Health Science Fit In?

The past decade has witnessed substantial mounting interest in "big data": the collection and analysis of vast points of information on individuals. The promise of big data from transformative applications to population health has been heralded; comprehensive biological information combined with high-quality bioinformatics on large samples of the population could, in theory, allow us to understand better who is at risk for disease and who responds to treatment, and allow us to develop better technologies for tracking and surveillance of health information (Hood and Flores 2012, Roski et al. 2014).

Although the exact amount of information that forms a "big" data set versus a "small" one remains ambiguous, scholars have increasingly described big data using three Vs (Roski et al. 2014, Mooney et al. 2015): variety (combining data from many different sources), volume (collecting many thousands of pieces of information for the data set), and velocity (rapid analysis in real-time using computer-generated algorithms).

In the field of health, big data have most often arrived in the form of high-volume data. The era of ever-increasing "-omics" fields (genomics, transcriptomics, proteomics, epigenomics, enviromics, and so on) has created a large amount of data resources on individual biological profiles at relatively low costs. Such vast arrays of data are proving to be successful in targeting cancer therapies based on genotypic variation (Jiang and Liu 2015). Researchers can analyze the genetic architecture of hundreds of thousands of study participants, conducting thousands upon thousands of statistical tests and procedures to determine how genetic sequencing increases our risk for diseases. These high-volume data have led to both mathematical and philosophical discussions about the role of traditional Fisherian–style statistical testing when data are amassed at such a volume and statistical tests run into the millions (McCarthy et al. 2008). New technologies have necessitated innovation in bioinformatics and biostatistics to redefine what it means to have a "finding," and have challenged our notions of the basic foundations of experimental paradigms of science. For example, classic experimental paradigms operate from a platform in which hypotheses are derived from theories and are then tested and falsified. In the era of high-volume -omics data, there is a movement toward hypothesis generation or data mining techniques that are purportedly atheoretical.

Current big data techniques often represent a relationship between researchers and private industry. For example, Google and its parent company Alphabet are at the forefront of championing how vast amounts of data might be able to transform population health. In addition to using technology aimed at developing better disease treatments and tracking, researchers are aiming to use data to develop our knowledge about causes of disease with the explicit goal of lengthening the average life span of humans. In 2015, the long-time director of the National Institute of Mental Health resigned from his position to take on a central role in developing new data technologies through Google X with the goal of better diagnosis and treatment of mental health problems using big data analytic techniques (Insel 2015). Although it remains to be seen how big data and technology will shape population health, there is certainly excitement in the field about developing new technology.

Although the introduction of big data in our population health armamentarium has occasioned some very reasonable concerns (Hoffman and Podgurski 2013), for the purposes of this book we note that, regardless of the size, scope, and speed of data acquisition and analysis, the foundational principles of population health science articulated here can guide the questions asked of big data warehouses, the direction taken by the science that improves the lives of populations, and the policy implications of working with big data resources. Regardless of the millions of points of biological data collected on individuals' risk for disease occurrence, the structural forces that drive housing, nutrition, poverty, access to resources, and education are likely to shape fundamentally how health is distributed across populations. It remains likely that many causes of incidence across populations are not the same as the causes of cases within populations, and such causes of incidence are likely distributed unequally across populations. Concerns about equity and efficiency and about appropriate ROI remain alive, well, and central to the utility—or potential lack thereof—of big data resources. To be sure, understanding how social, political, and interpersonal forces affect biology is a critical part of our task as population health scientists. Big data have the potential to enrich approaches informed by multilevel or life course perspectives. For example, real-time information on neighborhood factors, traffic patterns, and environmental risks have the potential to provide more rigorous assessments of the social environment than ever before (Ferreira et al. 2013). This remains, however, just one part of our mission, and it is critical that we, as population health scientists, shape the discourse around uses of big data, ensuring technology and excitement do not drive the questions asked, but rather improve our ability to answer them. To this end, we suggest the principles of population health science can guide these ever-increasing conversations, always reminding ourselves that prevention of disease is preferable to treatment, and we would do well to maximize our ROI by focusing resources on understanding preventive strategies that optimize health across the life course. We discussed throughout this book that, for example, early education and interventions early in life can have compounded returns to health throughout life. Using big data to uncover the factors that promote health early in life may be a lens through which to combine technology and data resources with a principled examination of our values.

3.0 Is Precision Medicine Antithetical or Complementary to Population Health Science Goals?

The promise of big data revolutionizing science and clinical care is linked to the rise of personalized and precision medicine (referred to here as *precision medicine*) heralding a new way in which clinical care will be delivered.

Broadly, precision medicine is a framework in which treatment decisions are customized to personal characteristics of patients, including biological information about the genome and exome, as well as phenotypic characteristics of symptoms, medical history, lifestyle, and other data points. This framework has already proved to be successful in many areas of clinical practice, including oncology (Roychowdhury and Chinnaiyan 2014), cystic fibrosis (Eckford et al. 2012), and other fields. Rare diseases that were previously often misdiagnosed are now diagnosed with better accuracy (Petrovski et al. 2015). Such precision medicine tools are often based on big data resources, and increasing calls from stakeholders in health encourage the further development of such resources to expand precision medicine approaches across a wide variety of health outcomes (Collins and Varmus 2015). Yet, the incorporation of precision medicine into a population health framework faces mathematical and conceptual challenges (Bayer and Galea 2015). This does not obviate a role for precision medicine in population health science thinking, but it militates for a careful engagement with precision medicine informed by the principles articulated here and the elevation of population concerns above all others.

Confronting mathematical reality first, a central goal of prediction is strong accuracy of individual predicted risk. In the literature on precision medicine, a common refrain is that such techniques will allow us to accurately predict who will get a particular disease, and will provide us with tools to identify risk factors that can be mitigated for prevention (Hood and Flores 2012). Yet, as we demonstrated in Chapter 10, the precision of such prediction is bounded by the factors that interact with those factors in the predictive model, and such factors likely vary across populations. This is consistent with our foundational principle of population health science that causes of differences in population health are not necessarily causes of differences in individual health. In fact, for most common diseases that affect population health, genomic and other biological predictors within populations are often poor discriminators of which individuals will develop disease, unless those genomic and other biological factors have an extraordinarily strong association with disease risk. Furthermore, stochastic factors likely underlie much of the individual differences in disease onset (Smith 2011). Thus, it is unlikely that precision medicine will be able to predict disease incidence risk strongly and accurately; and even if a predictive model is accurate in one population, it is likely to differ in accuracy across populations. This strongly suggests that precision medicine would benefit from a shift away from claims of individual prediction toward engagement with mechanistic processes, complementing both clinical disease and our understanding through which these conditions manifest as the health of individuals within populations.

Conceptually, we have focused much attention in this book on the central role prevention plays in population health. When we look back at factors that improved lives in the population dramatically in the past century, few have been personalized, or precise. We know vaccines do little good for the majority of individuals who get them, because they never would have gotten the disease in the first place. Car crashes remain relatively rare, but almost all states in the US have at least some form of mandatory seat belt laws. Clean air acts restrict the rights of individuals to smoke where and when they want, for the potential benefit of nonsmokers who may or may not be in the vicinity. These examples fall into the prevention paradox: that most people will not benefit from prevention efforts, and that large numbers of individuals who will not benefit still need to participate for population health to be maximized. Population health, then, is achieved when we decide collectively that we will change for the good of all, not for the benefit of any individual. How does this relate to precision medicine? Our ethos as a health community dictates the focus of our scholarship. We are increasing the technical capacity to understand the biology of disease with the potential to tailor treatments to specific genetic and other molecular sequences of the individual, which has proved the potential of transformative medicine. In the wake of these transformations in care, we should ensure our resources are equally balanced in promoting preventive efforts that are not individual and, in fact, may not benefit most individuals.

We framed this section as a question—is precision medicine antithetical or complementary to population health science?—and the answer to this question remains to be seen. Precision medicine is clearly an innovative and necessary step in clinical medicine and treatment. Yet, gains in precision medicine have been seen predominately for rare diseases for which underlying genetic causes and/or genomic markers are strongly determinant of disease phenotype. Thus, the role for precision medicine in population health is a difficult one to define, given that prevention for promotion of population health is key, and population health is not about individuals per se, but rather about population distributions made up of individuals. Decades of advances in population health science have shown us the answers to pressing population problems are found, paradoxically, by focusing explicitly not on individuals, but rather on populations. Consider, for example, heart disease and stroke. Despite dramatic declines in outcomes such as heart disease and stroke during the past century, such outcomes remain among the leading causes of death in the United States. The question for population health science is: How can we now progress to prevent such deaths, given the already vast improvements in the outcome that have been made through smoking cessation, dietary changes, and improvement in clinical care and management? We know heart disease and stroke are patterned socially, affect those in the lowest socioeconomic strata more than others, and are patterned geographically, as well, in ways that cannot be driven by biology. In a world of limited resources, should we invest our intellectual efforts and finances in pursuing biological markers of stroke risk or in improving conditions for low-income individuals, beginning in childhood, and supporting education and mobility throughout life? Of course, we should probably do both. However, and importantly, the actual number of scientists and dollars focusing on one versus the other is certainly not distributed equitably. To the extent that precision medicine overlooks the factors that cause population health, we must confront whether an unremitting investment in such biomedical approaches to detecting and treating disease will distract from achieving population health goals that would benefit millions with relatively more limited investment.

In sum, both prevention science and population health are concerned explicitly with the goal of improving health. Ample evidence throughout decades and even centuries has demonstrated the health of populations is determined centrally by investment in the macrosocial factors that drive the health of populations and by attention to prevention efforts that aim to improve the health of populations. As with all we have discussed in this book, tackling these issues is about our ability to understand, and eventually act on, the drivers of population health. We know that transforming population health rests on multilevel and life course approaches that combine a commitment to macrosocial determinants with an understanding of the mechanisms that link these determinants to health. Insofar as precision medicine can help do the latter, without compromising the former, the health of populations can indeed benefit from the emergence of precision medicine. It shall be to our collective detriment if precision medicine, however, distracts and detracts from our efforts to identify the complex causes that ultimately shape population health.

4.0 Can Population Approaches Inform Brain Imaging and Neuroscience?

As with other emerging areas of science described in this chapter, our ability to peer inside the human brain has progressed rapidly during the past 20 years. Functional magnetic resource imaging (fMRI) has allowed for an unparalleled ability to understand the structure and function of brain regions under different conditions, and the role of brain activity in social bonding, memory, and brain plasticity throughout the life course. In almost every area of research, understanding the effects of exposures on the brain, and the effects of brain structure and function on health and disease are fast becoming a reality. Reflecting the growing interest in understanding the human brain, the National Institutes of Health in 2015 committed $85,000,000 to increasing high-quality research aimed at understanding brain structure and function, as well as developing new technologies to treat brain disorders such as traumatic brain injury and epilepsy. Samples that include neuroimaging components are being increasingly collected on larger and larger cohorts of children, adolescents, and adults, in hope that, through understanding how the brain works, we can improve diagnosis, treatment, and etiological understanding of mechanisms.

The developing technologies in neuroscience are providing novel insights into the processes through which macrosocial determinants of health become embedded in individual health outcomes. Our understanding of the way in which the central macrosocial determinants of health such as poverty, discrimination, and education become embedded biologically to influence health and longevity is increasing rapidly as well (Khoury et al. 2012, Krieger 2012, Sheridan and McLaughlin 2014). Studies from large samples of children, for example, have demonstrated that children raised in poverty or social isolation manifest both structural and functional changes in brain activity at very young ages (McLaughlin et al. 2014), and such changes persist into adolescence and adulthood (McLaughlin and Hatzenbuehler 2009). These studies provide generalizations about processes through which context-specific exposures may influence health through biological imprinting, and create an evidence base for action with specific phenotypic outcomes to test potential interventions.

Yet, the science of brain imaging has not caught up to the science of sampling populations. Often, samples are selected specifically for certain characteristics, or based on those willing to submit to long protocols, which may be nonrepresentative of the general populations to which preventive interventions based on the results would be applied. Although the cost of imaging often precludes very large samples of individuals from populations, such costs are decreasing and the need for population-based samples is being increasingly recognized (Falk et al. 2013). Approaches to the study of the human brain that incorporate population health principles would increase the utility of this burgeoning field, including recognizing the causal architecture that underlies brain structure and function changes, how such architecture may change throughout the life course. These issues of representation and causal architecture array in a complex grid that should be theorized before data collection, and incorporated into analytic techniques. Understanding causal architecture requires recognizing the social and political context from which subjects are drawn, as well as hypothesizing explicitly how results and distributions of exposures may differ across different populations. In sum, a neuroscientific approach to the study of the social environment is an exciting avenue to achieving population health goals, and such approaches combined with epidemiological sampling that attends to population health principles could provide a marriage of techniques and theories that will provide an exciting benchmark for science in the decades to come.

5.0 Conclusion

Imagine a typical interaction between a patient, complaining of chest pain, and a doctor 20 or 50 years from now. What are the questions that will be asked and answered? On one hand, we could envision a future in which vast amounts of biological data predict the probability the patient has a number of clinical conditions and, using information about the patient's genome, exome, microbiome, and clinical history, suggest a course of action. But, we could also imagine a future in which the questions asked include how her neighbors are doing, what financial stress she is feeling, whether she has anxiety or mood problems, and whether her housing is secure. Which of these sets of questions is more technologically innovative? We suggest, provocatively perhaps, the latter. The latter set of questions may indeed hold the promise for health and wellness, and a research program that confronts the structural forces that place individuals at risk, creates distributions of health and disease unequally across socially defined groups, and focuses on embedding biological pathways within social interactions that develop and perpetuate across the life course and across generations, could be a call to action for population health as the science that creates and maintains healthy populations.

Population health science has a critical role in the ongoing developments in scientific innovation across big data bioinformatics techniques, precision medicine, and advances in understanding brain circuitry and function. Our role is to embed in these promising and potentially transformative technologies an understanding of our foundational principles, and ensure the way in which questions are asked and answered aligns with our value system. We fully expect and embrace that in the coming decades there will be better data, better techniques, and better understanding of biological systems. We argue, however, that none of these will replace the centrality of population approaches to understanding and improving health distributions. Our goal in writing this text is to provide population health scholars with a solid foundation in our understanding of health distributions and their causes that can then be applied to the transformative research across all areas of science, keeping an eye toward population health equity, efficiency in improving population health, and consequential questioning toward a science that matters.

6.0 References

Bayer, R., and S. Galea. (2015). Public health in the precision-medicine era. *N Engl J Med* **373**(6): 499–501.

Collins, F. S., and H. Varmus. (2015). A new initiative on precision medicine. *N Engl J Med* **372**(9): 793–795.

Eckford, P. D., C. Li, M. Ramjeesingh, and C. E. Bear. (2012). Cystic fibrosis transmembrane conductance regulator (CFTR) potentiator VX-770 (Ivacaftor) opens the defective channel gate of mutant CFTR in a phosphorylation-dependent but ATP-independent manner. *J Biol Chem* **287**(44): 36639–36649.

Falk, E. B., L. W. Hyde, C. Mitchell, J. Faul, R. Gonzalez, M. M. Heitzeg, et al. (2013). What is a representative brain? Neuroscience meets population science. *Proc Natl Acad Sci U S A* **110**(44): 17615–17622.

Ferreira, N., J. Poco, H. T. Vo, J. Freire, and C. T. Silva. (2013). Visual exploration of big spatio-temporal urban data: a study of New York City taxi trips. *IEEE Trans Vis Comput Graph* **19**(12): 2149–2158.

Hoffman, S., and A. Podgurski. (2013). The use and misuse of biomedical data: is bigger really better? *Am J Law Med* **39**(4): 497–538.

Hood, L., and M. Flores. (2012). A personal view on systems medicine and the emergence of proactive P4 medicine: predictive, preventive, personalized and participatory. *N Biotechnol* **29**(6): 613–624.

Insel, T. (2015). *Farewell*. NIMH director's blog. Available: http://www.nimh.nih.gov/about/director/2015/farewell.shtml.

Jiang, P., and X. S. Liu. (2015). Big data mining yields novel insights on cancer. *Nat Genet* **47**(2): 103–104.

Khoury, M. J., M. L. Gwinn, R. E. Glasgow, and B. S. Kramer. (2012). A population approach to precision medicine. *Am J Prev Med* **42**(6): 639–645.

Krieger, N. (2012). Methods for the scientific study of discrimination and health: an ecosocial approach. *Am J Public Health* **102**(5): 936–944.

McCarthy, M. I., G. R. Abecasis, L. R. Cardon, D. B. Goldstein, J. Little, J. P. Ioannidis, et al. (2008). Genome-wide association studies for complex traits: consensus, uncertainty and challenges. *Nat Rev Genet* **9**(5): 356–369.

McLaughlin, K. A., and M. L. Hatzenbuehler. (2009). Mechanisms linking stressful life events and mental health problems in a prospective, community-based sample of adolescents. *J Adolesc Health* **44**(2): 153–160.

McLaughlin, K. A., M. A. Sheridan, and H. K. Lambert. (2014). Childhood adversity and neural development: deprivation and threat as distinct dimensions of early experience. *Neurosci Biobehav Rev* **47**: 578–591.

Mooney, S. J., D. J. Westreich, and A. M. El-Sayed. (2015). Commentary: epidemiology in the era of big data. *Epidemiology* **26**(3): 390–394.

Petrovski, S., V. Shashi, S. Petrou, K. Schoch, K. M. McSweeney, R. S. Dhindsa, et al. (2015). Exome sequencing results in successful riboflavin treatment of a rapidly progressive neurological condition. *Cold Spring Harb Mol Case Stud* **1**: a000257.

Roski, J., G. W. Bo-Linn, and T. A. Andrews. (2014). Creating value in health care through big data: opportunities and policy implications. *Health Aff* **33**(7): 1115–1122.

Roychowdhury, S., and A. M. Chinnaiyan. (2014). Translating genomics for precision cancer medicine. *Annu Rev Genomics Hum Genet* **15**: 395–415.

Shaikh, A. R., A. J. Butte, S. D. Schully, W. S. Dalton, M. J. Khoury, and B. W. Hesse. (2014). Collaborative biomedicine in the age of big data: the case of cancer. *J Med Internet Res* **16**(4): e101.

Sheridan, M. A., and K. A. McLaughlin. (2014). Dimensions of early experience and neural development: deprivation and threat. *Trends Cogn Sci* **18**(11): 580–585.

Smith, G. D. (2011). Epidemiology, epigenetics and the 'gloomy prospect': embracing randomness in population health research and practice. *Int J Epidemiol* **40**(3): 537–562.

Index

accumulation of risk, 54f, 57–58, 59t
alcohol consumption level of select drinking groups, 74, 75f
alcohol-related consequences, macrosocial determinants of, 74–76

Bernand, Claude, 8–9
"big data," population health science and the rise of, 192–94
blood pressure. *See* hypertension; systolic blood pressure
body mass index (BMI). *See also* high-risk and population interventions/approaches; hypertension; obesity
    calculating, 158, 174
    high, 174, 175
brain imaging, population approaches informing, 197–99

car accidents, alcohol-related fatal, 75, 76f
cardiovascular disease. *See* coronary heart disease
causal architecture approach, 90–92
    implications for, 92–94
    understanding the impact of prevalent vs. rare causes mathematically, 99–104

causal inference, 14
    in population health science, 21–23
causal structure of disease, 147–48
causal thinking at the individual level, 15–19, 19f
causation, 14, 21–23
    conceptualized at the population level, 18–21, 20f
    population health
    quantitative examples of, 29–37
    when between- and within-population causes are distinct and dependent, 33–37
    when between- and within-population causes are distinct and independent, 30–33
cause, defined, 16–17
causes
    of cases within populations vs. incidence across populations, 25–29
    co-occurrence of, and their impact on population health science assessment, 105–6
    multiple, 16
    nature of, 14–15
    population health science approach to studying causes by focusing on what matters most, 89–90

causes (*Cont.*)
  of population health variation
    across the life course, 49, 52–58, 59*t*
    multilevel, 46–49, 47*f*, 48*f*, 50–52*b*
chains of risk, 54*f*, 56–57, 59*t*
cognitive ability, and understanding
    differing causal effects across
    populations, 102–4, 104*t*
coronary heart disease (CHD), 50–52*b*
  age-adjusted mortality rates from,
    50, 51*f*
"correlation is not causation," 23
critical/sensitive periods, 53–56, 54*f*, 59*t*
curve-shifting population health
    approach, 75

diethylstilbestrol (DES), 55
disability-adjusted life years (DALYs),
    113–16, 122, 123*f*, 124, 132, 133*f*,
    134, 134*f*
discounting rates, 121–22
disease. *See also* causes; health problems
  at the population level, 7–9
drug use, intravenous (IV), 70–72, 115

efficiency. *See* equity and efficiency
environment, unhealthy. *See* unhealthy
    environment
epidemiology, 86
epistemology of science, 5
equity and efficiency
  balancing, through high-risk and
    population interventions, 171–73
  nature of, 129–32
  and our value system as population
    health scientists, 138–39
  in population health, 132–35
  in population health science, examples
    of, 135–37
  tradeoffs between, 137–38
  when they are not in conflict, 137–38
exposure. *See also* ubiquitous exposures

shifting exposure prevalence
    across geographic space and
    time, 106–7
external validity, 93

genetic endowment, 103–4
genetic influences on cognitive ability,
    102–3, 104*t*
genetic (risk) variant, 145–48, 152, 153
genetic vulnerability, 28
  to obesity, 91, 159–62, 160*t*, 164*f*, 165,
    166, 168

health
  conceptualized on continua, 7–11,
    10*t*, 11*t*
  at the population level, 7–9
health disparities in U.S., macrosocial
    determinants of, 72–74
health inequalities. *See also* inequality
  gaining overall population health
    while creating, 134*f*, 134–35
health inequity. *See also* inequity
  gaining overall population health
    while increasing, 133*f*, 133–34
health problems. *See also* disease
  conceptualized on continua, 9–11,
    10*t*, 11*t*
heart disease. *See* coronary heart disease
hidden costs and consequences, 124–26
high-risk and population interventions/
    approaches
  the analytic approach, 174–78
  balancing equity and efficiency
    through, 171–73
  comparing, 40–43, 41*f*
high-risk groups. *See also* risk
  focusing on, 37–38
high-risk strategy, defined, 38
horizontal equity, 132–33, 136, 137
hypertension, prevalence of, 178–79, 181–83.
    See also systolic blood pressure

effects of interventions on population distributions of SBP and, 181–89
high-risk prevention interventions, 178–79, 180t, 181, 185–89
population prevention, 181

individual level, causal thinking at the, 15–19, 19f
individual-level variation. *See also* causes: of cases within populations vs. incidence across populations
vs. population-level variation, 18–21
process of explaining, 18
individual motivation, 159–62, 163t, 164t, 165–68
inequality. *See also* health inequalities
defined, 129, 130
vs. inequity, 129–30
inequity. *See also* health inequity
defined, 130
vs. inequality, 129–30
interaction, prediction of disease in the presence of, 149, 150f, 151f, 152–54
internal validity, 93
interventions. *See also* high-risk and population interventions/approaches
impact over time, 118–21
assessing, 121–22
and return on health, 122, 123f, 124
intravenous (IV) drug use, 70–72, 115

Let's Move!, 158
life course approaches to population health science, 49, 52–58, 59t
life course models and approaches to population health science, 58, 59t

macrosocial determinants
of alcohol-related consequences, 74–76
of health, and implications for population health science, 78–80
macrosocial factors, 69
as drivers of population health distributions, examples of, 72–78
miasmatic thinking, 48–49
mortality, income inequality and, 69–72, 70t, 71t
motor vehicle crash fatalities, alcohol-related, 75, 76f
multilevel causes of population health variation, 46–49, 47f, 48f, 50–52b

neuroscience, population approaches informing, 197–99

obesity, 157–59. *See also* high-risk and population interventions/approaches; hypertension
causal structure, 159–66, 160t
a population health science approach to, 166–68
opportunity cost, 122

paradigms, 5
shifting, 93–94
Pareto efficiency, 131–32
personalized and precision medicine. *See* precision medicine
population attributable risk proportion (PARP), 161, 162, 164f, 165, 166
population density, 46–47
population health as a continuum, 8
examples of, 9–11
population health science. *See also specific topics*
definition and nature of, 1, 4–6
foundational principles of, *xiii*, 2, 7, 8b, 21b, 37, 39, 42b, 62b, 72b, 106b, 121b, 138b, 154b, 187–89

population health science (*Cont.*)
    combined with rapidly developing science, 191–92
  and other sciences, 4–5
population health thinking, dangers of, 48–49
population health variation, dynamic interactions and, 59–62
population level, health and disease at the, 7–9
population-level variation, 18
  vs. individual-level variation, 18–21
populations
  a different set of causes can produce the same causal effect across, 101–2
  nature of, 4
  the same set of causes can produce different causal effects across, 100–101
  understanding differing causal effects across, 102–4
precision medicine, 194
  as antithetical vs. complementary to population health science goals, 194–97
prediction of disease when there is interaction, 149, 150*f*, 151*f*, 152–54
predictive medicine for population health, limits of, 146–53
predictive validity, assessing, 142–45
predictive value
  limitations of translating population measures to individualized prediction, 145–46
  positive, 142–45
prevention. *See also specific topics*
  the value of, 118–21
prevention paradox, 42, 43, 118, 188, 196
prevention strategies for population health, 37

comparing high-risk vs. population approaches, 40–43, 41*f*
focusing on high-risk groups, 37–38
focusing on the population, 39–40
preventive medicine
  defined, 6
  public health, population health science, and, 6
public health
  defined, 6
  preventive medicine, population health science, and, 6

quality-adjusted life years (QALYs), 113, 116–18

racial discrimination, 73–74
racial segregation, 79
return on investment (ROI), 111–12
  for health, 112–18
returns on health investments, measuring end points in, 113
risk. *See also* high-risk and population interventions/approaches
  accumulation of, 54*f*, 57–58, 59*t*
  chains of, 54*f*, 56–57, 59*t*
risk factor approaches to the study of disease
  vs. causal architecture, 90–91, 91*f*
  limits of, 86–88
  moving beyond, 92
risk factor epidemiology, 86
risk factors, defined, 86
Rose, Geoffrey A., 2–3, 25, 26, 29, 43, 94, 167
  on the difference between understanding sick individuals and sick populations, 28
  on high risk approach, 172, 187
  on prevention paradox, 42, 188
  The Strategy of Preventive Medicine, 2, 3

science
 combining foundational principles with rapidly developing, 191–92
 epistemology of, 5
 nature of, 4
 philosophy of, 5
sciences, population health science and other, 4–5
secondary prevention, 172, 173
 of hypertension, 173, 176–79, 180*t*, 181, 182*t*, 184, 185*t*, 186, 188
sensitive periods. *See* critical/sensitive periods
shifting the curve, 39
social norms as macrosocial determinants, 76–78
Strategy of Preventive Medicine, The (Rose), 2, 3
structural factors, 49
structural forms of discrimination, 73–74
systolic blood pressure (SBP), 173. *See also* hypertension
 distribution of, 174, 175*f*, 178, 179*f*, 181–83
 prevention strategies and, 179, 179*f*, 181, 183*f*

time preference, 122
traffic fatalities, alcohol-related, 75, 76*f*

ubiquitous causes, 25
ubiquitous exposures and population health, 68–72
ubiquity, metaphor for, 68–69, 69*f*
unhealthy environment, 160*t*, 160–62, 163*t*, 164*t*, 165–68
 defined, 159
unintended costs and consequences, 124–26
utero environment as critical period, 55

validity, internal and external, 93
vertical equity, 132–33

years lost as a result of disability (YLD), 114–15
years of life lost (YLL), 114, 115